Curriculum Revolution: Reconceptualizing Nursing E

Pub. No. 15-2280

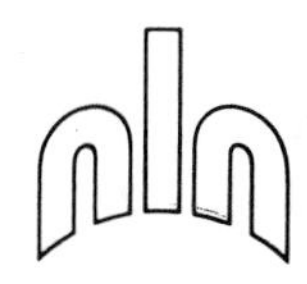

National League for Nursing • New York

ISBN 0-88737-442-5

Manufactured in the United States of America

Contributors

Em Olivia Bevis, MA, RN, FAAN
Nursing Educational Consultant
Adjunct Research Professor
Georgia Southern College
Statesboro, Georgia

Peggy L. Chinn, PhD, RN, FAAN
Professor of Nursing
State University of New York at Buffalo
Buffalo, New York

Gloria M. Clayton, EdD, RN
Associate Professor
School of Nursing
Medical College of Georgia
Athens, Georgia

Nancy L. Diekelmann, PhD, RN, FAAN
Professor
School of Nursing
University of Wisconsin–Madison
Madison, Wisconsin

Sister Rosemary Donley, PhD, RN, FAAN
President, National League for Nursing
Executive Vice President
The Catholic University of America
Washington, DC

Barbara A. Hedin, PhD, RN
Assistant Professor
Teachers College, Columbia University
New York, New York

Carol A. Lindeman, PhD, RN, FAAN
Dean
School of Nursing
Oregon Health Sciences University
Portland, Oregon

Clair E. Martin, PhD, RN
Dean and Professor
Nell Hodgson Woodruff School of Nursing
Emory University
Atlanta, Georgia

Patricia Moccia, PhD, RN
Vice President, Education and Accreditation
National League for Nursing
New York, New York

Joyce P. Murray, MSN, RN
Associate Professor
Department of Nursing
Georgia Southern College
Statesboro, Georgia

Verle Waters, MA, RN
Assistant Dean
Health and Science
Ohlone College
Freemont, California

Contents

Preface

The word curriculum comes from the Latin, meaning race course. As the 1980s come to a close, nursing is running at a sprinter's speed. Never before has there been so much to do in such a limited time; never has nursing had to deal with so many outside forces that seem nearly insurmountable.

Those of us who are running this race are fully prepared for the challenge, yet unlike most competitions, we would all like to finish at the same time—everyone should be a winner and nobody should be lagging behind. We need to make certain that we are all running the same race for the same purpose. Naturally, the best way to accomplish this is through effective communication.

The type of exchange which characterized the presentations at the National League for Nursing's Fifth National Conference on Nursing Education in 1988 which comprise this volume reveals the broadening scope of issues affecting nursing's present and future. Although each author explores a different topic, one theme appears throughout: Nursing does not exist in a vacuum—it consistently affects and is affected by society.

Rather than passively accepting the conditions society imposes, nursing leaders are reconceptualizing their and other's approaches to both theory and curriculum. Such issues as feminism, the changing profile of today's nurses, innovations in clinical teaching, as well as overall economic and social trends are forcing health care to become more reality-based than ever before. We simply cannot address today's concerns with yesterday's theories and expect positive results.

As modern curriculum builders, we are anxious to implement change. Yet before improved admission criteria, program content, and job functions can be developed, our minds and spirits must be transformed. We invite you to hear our voices, discuss our ideas, but most importantly, to join the race, and be prepared for the challenge of your life.

1

Curriculum Revolution: Heeding the Voices of Change

Sister Rosemary Donley, PhD, RN, FAAN

In December of 1987, the nursing education community gathered in Philadelphia at the Fourth Nursing Education Conference to chart a course for a curriculum revolution in nursing. Some very innovative and even radical concepts were presented at that meeting. Everyone in attendance was inspired by a powerful mandate to create fundamental changes in the way we educate nurses— a mandate that called for a transformation of nursing curricula from a training model to a schema that would educate caring, critically thinking health care professionals.

The presenters developed compelling arguments to support the need for change, citing dramatic shifts in the health care system; the ill-effects of fee-for-service medicine on patients, nurses, and physicians; changing patterns in the nursing labor force; the new patient profile; the need for research and innovation in clinical teaching; and the need to broaden and enhance the humanistic aspects of nursing practice.

A year has passed since we heard those voices of change. Now we must move from concept to implementation, or, as Donald Schon says in his book *The Reflective Practitioner* (1983), from the high ground of abstract knowledge to the "messy," hands-on problem solving that comes when people try to make theory work in practice. According to Schon, it is this challenge which requires far greater knowledge and experience than the noble art of theory-building itself. Pressman and Wildavsky (1973), political scientists who are experts in the areas of federal legislative and budgetary processes, express the same reality—implementation is not easy.

Change of this magnitude is never simple. Revolutionizing the nursing curricula engages us in the complex and potentially dangerous task of moving forward with dramatic changes while preserving hard-earned successes and well-earned recognition. The transition from the safe ground of a clear-cut, objective, and highly refined training model to the ambiguous notion of health as human caring lacks the roadmap and cognitive surety of making simple, true and false choices. We are challenged because embarking on this course signals the beginning of a revolution that will never end—one in which we continually reexamine our curricula and the roles of students and teachers in light of new student populations, evolving health care systems, and a societal influx. We commit ourselves to ask essential questions again and again, and accept that no answer will be the final word.

Educators are challenged because we as well as our students will lack the assurance that we have defined and met the objective. But if we falter in our ambitious quest for change, we do a disservice—perhaps a gross injustice—to our profession, our students, and most significantly, those we are educated to care about. Our failure to risk change would be particularly noticeable at a time when people desperately need ethical and humanistic caregivers. As Pat Moccia reminded us last year in her address entitled, "Curriculum Revolution: An Agenda for Change," "every day, from moment to moment, nurses witness a society characterized by alienation and dehumanization as they become involved in the lives of the patients who come to their institutions and agencies seeking care, compassion, and help. Every day, nurses struggle to help a growing number of people whose lives are increasingly fragmented, constricted, and impoverished as a result of public and social policies" (Moccia, 1988, p. 53).

A recent story on the front page of the *Wall Street Journal* ("Dumping the Poor," 1988) graphically illustrates the urgency of our humanistic quest. The story examined the rash of "hospital dumping" of patients who are unable to pay their medical bills. The reporter recounted case after case of patients who were denied the most basic human care by the huge biomedical enterprise which we call the health care system. Among those cases was Terry Takewell, a 21-year-old diabetic from Tennessee who was brought to a nearby hospital after neighbors found him panting and drenched with sweat. A self-employed carpenter, Mr. Takewell had no health insurance and owed the hospital almost $10,000. His name was on a directive in the emergency room telling hospital staff members to alert their supervisors if he ever returned. Mr. Takewell was in a hospital bed when an administrator arrived; spoke with him briefly; then helped the patient to his feet and escorted him to the parking lot. Mr. Takewell's neighbors found him under a tree and took him home. He died shortly thereafter. The article concluded that, despite the presence of laws against it, some 250,000 patients are transferred from hospitals each year for purely economic reasons.

The voice of Mr. Takewell cries for professionals educated to care and create change in a complex health care system. Nurse educators must embrace a model of education which integrates moral reasoning and ethical values with technical expertise. It is only this mode of education that will prepare students to modify and rationalize situations such as those that engulfed Mr. Takewell.

John Dewey, one of our greatest educational theorists, spoke prophetically about similar issues more than 50 years ago. In his book, *Experience & Education* (1963), he asks why so many people look back upon their school years and wonder what became of the knowledge they were supposed to have amassed. To answer the question, he makes 2 points that bear directly on our quest for change.

> One trouble is that the subject-matter in question was learned in isolation; . . . It was segregated when it was acquired and . . . is so disconnected from the rest of experience that it is not available under the actual conditions of life. [When we ask] where has it gone to, the right answer is that it is still there in the special compartment in which it was originally stowed away.
>
> It is contrary to the laws of experience that learning of this kind should give genuine preparation. . . . What avail is it . . . If in the process the individual loses his own soul: loses his appreciation of things worth while, of the values to which these things are relative; if he loses desire to apply what he has learned and, above all, loses the ability to extract meaning from his future experiences as they occur?

These words add new meaning to the voices of change within nursing's curriculum revolution when they are heard in concert with other voices. We have elected a new president who defined his campaign by a promise of a kinder and gentler America. Many of us question how that phrase will influence policy, but that is not the issue.

The point is that voters responded to what the political and media experts behind the Bush campaign said they wanted to hear.

Americans elected George Bush and endorsed his tag as an "education president" who will work to instill moral values through education. Recasting our education programs on a philosophical foundation of humanism and of caring is what our curriculum revolution is all about.

We educators join our initiative with other voices for change. We witness the continuing greying of the population, as our over-65 population will reach the 13 percent mark by the year 2000 and 21 percent by the year 2030, when the baby boom generation reaches 65. (United States Bureau of the Census, 1989) Projections for the year 2040 estimate the number of people in nursing homes to be 4 times the number reported in 1980 (Mezey & Scanlon, 1988), and a disturbing report released recently indicated that 40 percent of the 15,000 nursing homes do not meet sanitary standards for handling food and 25 percent do not administer medication properly (Health Care Financing Administration, 1988). These statistics and reports are a powerful mandate for change in nursing education—a mandate to carefully consider the question, "What do elderly people need to be healthy—to maintain independence, autonomy, and cognitive, spiritual, emotional, and physical integrity—and how can we educate our students and ourselves to assist older people?"

Clearly responsibility to our elders demands a commitment from professional nursing to educate students to understand and manage the factors that create dependency—untreated illness; depression; poverty; social isolation; loss of mobility; memory loss; and diminished orientation to people, places, and things. We must plan for tomorrow's long-term care centers—nurse-run senior citizen apartment complexes, day care centers, respite care centers, and geriatric health clubs and clinics. Tomorrow's nursing homes have the potential to be similar to modern hospitals in that they will provide care and support to people whose conditions make care and treatment in the community impossible (Donley, 1988).

Coupled with all of this are the grim facts that hospitals continued to close their doors in greater numbers this year and no new hospitals opened in 1988. Arthur Anderson (1987) indicates that by 1990, 700 hospitals will shut down. Hospital admissions are falling because the medical model of care has grown unacceptably expensive and increasingly ill-suited to the needs of older, chronically ill people. Society is asking nursing education to emphasize caring, as well as curing. More patients and clients will seek care outside hospital walls. Our educational systems have linked learning about the experience of illness and treatment to the hospital. This assumption needs to be reexamined as we move forward with our curriculum revolution. It is our job as educators to shape curricula that will prepare nurses to assume primary care and case management roles in all care settings.

There are other voices for change: the growing number of drug users and homeless people whose lifestyles jeopardize their health and lives. We do not address substance abuse in our curricula—yet drugs and the violence associated with drug-addicted and alcoholic lifestyles deplete our country of human resources and have made sections of American cities virtual wastelands.There is widespread evidence that the drug problem has escalated to new heights this year, with an alarming surge nationwide in the quantity and use of homemade amphetamines known as speed. Instead of replacing cocaine and crack, this potentially lethal substance stimulates more drug use, and emergency rooms report dramatic increases in the number of people with drug-induced psychoses. Law officials are dismayed by its rapid spread.

More statistics which cannot be ignored are those describing the growth of the number of homeless. The Committee on Health Care for Homeless People (1988) reports that some 735,000 Americans are homeless on any given night, while 1.3 to 2 million people will be homeless for one night or more in a year. If the Robert Wood Johnson data on health care of the homeless are accurate, homeless people will respond to health care that is centered around understanding and human interaction (Wright & Weber, 1987).

The fact that our students suffer reality shock—the gap between the nursing of the education world and the nursing of the practice world—is not surprising. A new National League for Nursing survey (in press) includes a broad range of questions about educational and on-the-job experiences of newly licensed nurses. One message that came through with disturbing frequency is expressed by a BSN graduate: "My clinical experiences in school were nowhere close to those I am experiencing now in practice . . . I am saddened that in less than one year my thoughts and feelings about nursing have changed so drastically."

Let's listen to another voice. The recent report of a national panel of medical professionals stated that American medical education has fallen out of step with society's needs. This panel calls for dramatic changes in the way medical schools admit, train, and test students. According to the panel's findings, the nation's 127 medical schools are "preparing doctors for medicine of the past," especially in doctor–patient relationships. There should be less emphasis placed on exams and more on the ability of doctors to work competently and sensitively with patients (Rogers, 1988). If poverty, aging, substance abuse, and homelessness were not enough, we hear the voices of the numerous people who are sick with AIDS or worried about the presence of antibodies to the HIV virus in their blood. We are faced with the logistics of the revolution—the familiar problem of implementation. Where do we begin? How do we capture the active participation of the learner in the educational enterprise?

This is a critical point in the revolution. It comes first on any agenda for change. Doing this will not only help to design curricula that fully respect and make full use of the student experience in learning, but will engage students now, so that they may become partners in the revolution.

We can no longer imagine the teacher's role as that of information giver, as in Tyler-type technical behaviorism. As Em Olivia Bevis explains in her chapter on curriculum revolution, "The teacher's main purpose, beyond the minimal activity of insuring safety, is to provide the climate, the structure, and the dialogue to promote praxis. To design ways to engage the student in the mental processes of analysis . . . Until patterns are seen that provide paradigms for practice. . . . The teacher's role is to nurture the learner: to nurture the ethical ideal, to nurture the caring role. . . . [and] to interact with students as persons of worth, dignity, intelligence, and high scholarly standards" (Bevis, 1988, p. 46).

We must not overthrow one system with another to take its place. Everyone is changed in a revolution, which is why we must be careful not to dismiss the Tyler model in its entirety. We cannot blame the Tyler rationale or any organizing framework for all of nursing's curriculum trouble. It has had a positive impact on the quality of nursing education. The strict insistence on measurable objectives backed by the force of law, custom, and accreditation has produced an organized, evaluation-oriented system that provides services of reliable quality. Nurse educators monitor and police themselves with a sense of responsibility and commitment to public trust. That is not found in medical, legal, technical, or business models of education.

Accreditation cannot be ignored in any curriculum revolution. Some educators see a conflict in a curriculum revolution when accreditation criteria are modeled on the Tyler rationale. As we wrote when preparing the standards for accreditation, nursing accreditation responds to those who are free and open, make their voices heard, take part in the meeting of the councils, conduct site visits and participate in board of review. Accreditation criteria have evolved. They will continue to evolve and change. It is in forums such as these meetings where the process of change begins. But as Dewey observes, "We have to stop, look, and listen," whenever we propose dramatic changes in education, whether it be in the curricula, in the accreditation policies, in interactions with students or in those quiet moments when we realize that we (the teachers-doers) must change.

This is not the first curriculum revolution on higher education. Like military strategists, we would be wise to study the successes and failures of other revolutions. In the last chapter in *Educating the Reflective Practitioner* (1987), Schon describes a small curriculum revolution at the Massachusetts Institute of Technology Department of Urban Studies and Planning. From 1981 to 1984, Schon was part of a small group that restructured the core curriculum for the master of city planning program. He describes a faculty of about 30 full-time members who valued research and practice, took teaching seriously but ranked it second to research and practice, and regarded administration as an "unavoidable and onerous duty." The student body was increasingly dissatisfied with the core curriculum; they found it fragmented and divorced from an understandable context. As students, they felt isolated from faculty members and believed they were being treated in core courses as though they had no prior knowledge.

Enter the revolution, which began quite predictably with a committee, but one with an interesting composition of members—three faculty members and *seven* first-year students from the program. Schon called the atmosphere of the committee meetings contentious. One student called them "a little scary," but the meetings provided the energy that every revolution requires.

The committee went public at the beginning, submitting ideas to students and faculty for inspection. One committee member said

"Everybody [was] in there. There was an extraordinary number of people . . . a democratic process which made a real effort to canvass . . . students and faculty."

Not surprisingly, the most important division of opinion arose between those who favored a "core" *that emphasized teaching students to think,* and those who favored a "core" *that gave priority to technical skills.* In the end, the committee proposed a conceptual approach to course content along with skill building sequences and practicums. They made some compromises on issues of "coherence versus flexibility" and the ways to give students greater access to faculty members. They allotted "time for reflection" in smaller groups, dealt with pass/fail grades, and recommended that controversial issues of the workplace be included as top priority.

I think you'll agree that the issues are strikingly familiar. Nurse educators are not the first to struggle with these concepts. In ancient Greece the tension was between the Acropolis and with the Agra. Schon stated that the group "paid attention to the process by which we tried to surface and resolve our conflicting ideas, and increasingly, over time, we thought of ourselves as engaged in an experiment in collective inquiry."

Did the curriculum revolution at MIT work? Yes, sort of, and not at all, says Schon. Some goals were fully realized, others only to a degree, and others not at all, and in the true spirit of the revolution, the new core continues to evolve.

But they did it, and we can take heart in the unexpected perk that benefitted everyone: new, powerful, and lasting sources of creative energy throughout the program.

I wish I could conclude by saying that with just a little careful planning and some extra time and effort we can make our curriculum revolution happen. But as seasoned educators we know what is before us.

However at those times when a little voice inside tells you to forget it all and return to the comfortable and familiar, listen to the stronger voices and consider the consequences of inaction. We need a kinder and gentler America. America deserves a health, not an illness care system that is held together, in the elegant words of Virginia Henderson, by nurses whose "hearts and heads and hands" can work as one.

Long live the revolution.

REFERENCES

Anderson, A., & American College of Health Care Executives. (1987). *The future of health care: Changes and choices.* Chicago: Arthur Anderson and Company.

Bevis, E. O. (1988). New directions for a new age. In *Curriculum revolution: Mandate for change* (pp. 27–52). New York: National League for Nursing.

Committee on Health Care for Homeless People. (1988). *Homelessness, health, and human needs.* Washington, DC: National Academy Press.

Dewey, J. (1963). *Experience and education.* New York: Macmillan.

Donley, Sr. R. (1988). Building nursing's platform for the long-term care debate. *Nursing and Health Care, 9*(6), 303–305.

Dumping the poor: Despite federal law, hospitals still reject sick who can't pay. (1988, November 29). *Wall Street Journal,* p. 1.

Health Care Financing Administration. (1988). *Medicare/Medicaid nursing home information.* Washington, DC: Author.

Mezey, M. D., & Scanlon, W. (1988). Registered nurses in nursing homes. In *Secretary's Commission on Nursing final report* (Vol. 2). Washington, DC: Department of Health and Human Services.

Moccia, P. (1988). Curriculum revolution: An agenda for change. In *Curriculum revolution: Mandate for change* (pp. 53–64). New York: National League for Nursing.

National League for Nursing. (in press). *Profiles of the newly licensed nurse.* New York: National League for Nursing.

Pressman, J., & Wildavsky, A. (1973). *Implementation.* Berkeley, CA: University of California Press.

Rogers, D. E. (1988). Clinical education and the doctor of tomorrow. In B. Gastel & D. E. Rogers (Eds.), *Proceedings of the Josiah Macy, Jr. Foundation National Seminar on Medical Education.* The New York Academy of Medicine.

Schon, D. (1983). *The reflective practitioner.* New York: Basic Books.

Schon, D. (1987). *Educating the reflective practitioner.* San Francisco: Jossey-Bass.

United States Bureau of the Census. (1989). *Projections of the population of the United States by age, sex, and race: 1988–2080* (Series P-25, No. 1018). Washington, DC: Author.

Wright, J. D., & Weber, E. (1987). *Homelessness and health.* Washington, DC: McGraw-Hill's Healthcare Information Center.

2

Feminist Pedagogy in Nursing Education

Peggy L. Chinn, PhD, RN, FAAN

Pedagogy is the art, science, or profession of teaching. Pedagogy, as an idea, is as old as education itself. However, those who teach and those who learn are most often unaware of what constitutes the particular pedagogy with which they are working.

PEDAGOGY WITHIN A PATRIARCHY

Pedagogy is something that is alive; it is a total package. It exists in the actions we take in the learning environment, the materials we use, how we use them, and the attitudes we convey. All teaching and learning encounters can be characterized by a pedagogy. Most pedagogies we use today are patriarchal or masculinist, in that they derive from ideas about how to teach and learn that come from a predominantly male experience of the world. The content that is identified as important to learn comes from the same source. The "authorities" and authoritative literature from whom we glean the specific content to be learned is almost always that of male authors, derived from male experience and views of the world. The skills that are thought of as useful to learn are identified because of their ultimate value in male-dominated social and political systems. The attitudes that are thought of as important to instill in students are identified as valuable for learning because they are the attitudes that serve us well in male-defined situations. The "logic" that is thought to characterize the educated mind is a logic of masculinist thinking.

Material from *Peace and Power: A Handbook of Feminist Process* (Second edition) is used with permission of the authors.

The institutions in which we do our teaching are patriarchal institutions, arranged in power-over hierarchies that diminish human experience, despite the educational philosophies of important humanist forefathers. The language that is used to describe existing pedagogies reflects assumptions and views of the world that derive from patriarchal ideologies and world views, which are seldom questioned (Spender, 1982). Consider examples such as:

- *Grades.* Alphabetical characters that are assigned a rank order and given numerical value that is multiplied and divided at will, and used for purposes of life-shattering consequence. One wonders, grades of what, for what end? Who benefits?
- *Teacher–student.* The "one" who knows and gives, the "other" who does not know and absorbs that which is given, preferably without questioning. Both are usually assumed to be male unless proven otherwise.
- *Lecture.* A one-way communication of pouring forth, declaring "truth"; the ultimate in expression of the syndrome "academentia" (Daly & Caputi, 1987). Usually based on knowledge set forth by male "authority," regardless of the gender of the lecturer.
- *Course.* The one appropriate path to knowledge, prescribed by institutions that charge a fee for taking the path, and measured in numbers of hours spent sitting in a specified room, in a specified chair.
- *Objectives.* The ultimate tautology—objectives are defined by the teacher, the giver of knowledge, as that which is worthy to know and learn, and it is the teacher who declares their achievement. This concept was conceived by male victims of logical thought. Usually achievement of these linguistic descriptors is measured by numerical signifiers, usually in examinations.
- *Examinations.* The "one" who truly "knows" places the "other" in a particularly uncomfortable and threatening situation, which is deemed all the better to "prove" whether the other "knows" anything at all.

Given these realities, a shift to feminist pedagogy is a radical shift. Pedagogically, there is nothing that can be taken for granted. Everything we do in preparing for the learning encounter, the content we plan, the language we use, the way we conduct ourselves, what we value, the attitudes we convey, the behaviors we nurture, the literature we draw on, the way we think about our purpose, what we hope to accomplish—everything—takes a dramatic shift into an entirely different realm (Weiler, 1988). For feminism itself is a dramatic shift in relation to the world as we now know it and experience it.

Feminism is valuing women, and all that is associated in our culture with women and women's experience. Feminist pedagogy derives from content that is viewed and experienced with women at the center. It draws on women's writings and other forms of women's accounts of their views and experience. (Note that women have been excluded from literary circles for centuries; therefore our literature is not limited to what is typically thought of as "literature".) It draws on skills that are central to women's experience. It nurtures attitudes that are valued in terms of women's realities. It draws on women's ways of thinking.

Feminist pedagogy can sometimes be seen as being in a dialectic relationship with masculinist pedagogy, but in my opinion, the two are not in a strictly dialectic posture with one another. Masculinist ideas and pedagogies have existed for centuries without a glimmer of concern for women's experience, realities, or views, even though they have been sustained and made possible by the material energy, scrubbing, feeding, and nurturing of countless women. Feminist ideas derive, in large part, from this very experience of supporting and making possible the masculinist world of reality. Therefore, a feminist view takes that reality into account. Feminist ideas consistently flow in a direction of healing splits in our experience and in our thinking, seeking to bring that together that can be, with that which is. Feminist methods are based on the premise that perceiving the whole leads to a fuller and richer understanding of what we know, and how we know it.

Sandra Harding (1987) has pointed out that "a feminist standpoint is not something anyone can have by claiming it, but an achievement. (A standpoint differs in this respect from a perspective.) To achieve a feminist standpoint one must engage in the intellectual and political struggle necessary to see nature and social life from the point of view of that disdained activity which produces women's social experiences instead of from the partial and perverse perspective available from the 'ruling gender' experience of men" (Harding, 1987, p. 185). This insight explains how feminist ideas can develop within the context of patriarchal institutions like schools and universities, and how we as teachers can do the political work of feminist pedagogy within those walls. As we do so, we experience the material realities of the intellectual and political struggle that are essential to achieving a feminist standpoint. We begin to consciously do what we know. As we act, we learn about a new way of being in the world.

PEDAGOGY, FEMINISM, AND NURSING

This is an extremely important undertaking for women who are nurses. The two ideas—pedagogy and feminism—have profound, indeed radical, meaning for nursing education. When we bring these two ideas together, we have a profound shift in the highly political process of education. In the context of nursing education, we begin to create a foundation for a profound shift in health care.

We begin to assume a questioning, skeptical stance toward everything that we have previously thought and known, and we become open to possibilities that we had never before taken seriously. The experience is transformative; it begins within. The shifts are both familiar and strange. Most of what we begin to experience are ways of being and doing that are familiar to everyone, particularly to women. However, at the same time they also feel strange because they are ways of thinking and being that have for our entire lives been devalued; and that we have worked to deny, compartmentalize, or see as somehow less than useful. These ways of thinking and doing do not exclude some of the possibilities that predominate in the masculinist world, which is why I sometimes find a dialectic view of these pedagogies to be less than useful. Rather, all possibilities are considered and questioned, but what remains constant is the fundamental commitment in relation to women and women's experience, and an ethic based on this perspective.

PEDAGOGY, PRAXIS, AND POWER

Feminist pedagogy is based on a feminist praxis. Feminist praxis incorporates thoughtful reflection and action that occur in synchrony toward the goal of transforming the world. The transformation that is sought is a vision that is grounded in feminist ethics and ideas about the way the world could be for all people. Central to feminist visions about the world as it could be is consciousness—full awareness that is based on a conviction that "I Know what I Do, and I Do what I Know" (Wheeler & Chinn, 1989).

Feminist praxis is concerned with power. Feminist praxis consciously rejects "power over" forms of power, but rather seeks personal empowerment and exercise of personal power in the world that leads to growth, transformation, unity, justice, and peace. How women experience power in our own lives (our own power or lack of it, or the powers of others over us) is central to the conceptions that have developed about power from a feminist perspective.

Power, and the closely related concept of empowerment, is therefore central to feminist pedagogy. Charlene Wheeler and I have conceptualized feminist forms of power in relation to group process and in relation to a teaching–learning experience. These feminist forms of power are derived from a perspective that values women and women's realities, along with women's concerns about how the world could be. These powers and some specific ways in which they are enacted in teaching and learning are:

Power of Process

Objectives, timeframes, and educational structures of evaluation may be used as tools that provide a structure from which to work, but they are not the focal point. The *process* is the important dimension, so that once the interaction begins the structure is *only* a tool and nothing more. *How* the interactions happen become the central focus, rather than a precise adherence to a prescribed content. Language is chosen as a tool to make the process possible, to create mental images that reduce the power imbalances of the institution and create new relationships. The process itself becomes part of the "text" for teaching and learning.

Power of Letting Go

All participants let go of old habits and ways in order to make room for personal and collective growth. Teachers let go of "power over" attitudes and ways of being; registrants let go of "tell me what to do" attitudes and ways of being. All participants move into ways of being that are personally empowering and that also nurture the empowerment of others.

Power of the Whole

Mutual help networks within the group are encouraged. Every individual is responsible to invest talents and skills for the interests of the group as a whole. Each participant, whether teacher or registrant, is accountable to the whole group for negotiating specific agendas, keeping the group informed as to absences, leaving early, arriving late, or initiating particular learning experiences.

Power of Collectivity

Each participant is taken into account in the group's planning-in-process. The group works to address the needs of learners who are moving into individual journeys where others may not be going. The needs of learners who are having specific struggles are addressed by the group in some way. Learners do not compete with one another; rather, the needs of all learners are acknowledged and addressed as equally valuable.

Power of Unity

Unity is viewed as coming from the expression of conflict and differing points of view so that the various points of view can be understood by all, and integrated into a richer and fuller appreciation of every individual. Learning is not merely accumulating the truths that are passed along by an authority, or accepting those ideas as "truth," but rather is an attitude of actively seeking to understand the possibilities of differing perspectives.

Power of Sharing

All participants enter the group with talents, skills, and abilities related to the education project, and actively engage in sharing their individual talents with the group. Teachers enter learning groups with previously developed capabilities that are shared according to the needs of the group and in consideration of the structure-as-tool. Registrants enter the group with personal talents, background, and experiences that are valued and shared. All participants enter the group as learners, open to what others can share.

Power of Integration

All dimensions of the situation are acknowledged to form a whole experience. Each individual's unique and self-defined needs for the learning experience are acknowledged and integrated into the process. The first portion of each gathering is used as a time for each individual to express her or his priorities, needs, and wishes for the gathering so that these can be integrated as a part of the process for that gathering.

Power of Nurturing

Each participant is respected fully and unconditionally, and treated as necessary and integral to the experience of the group. Learning activities and approaches are planned to nurture the gradual growth of new skills and abilities, assuring that every participant can be successful both in terms of the planned structure of the experience, and in terms of her or his individual needs.

Power of Intuition

The process that occurs, and the nature of what is addressed in the learning encounter depend as much on the experience of the moment as on any other factor. What emerges as important for the group to address in the moment is what happens. Letting go of what "ought" to happen is valued as a new skill that makes possible what will happen.

Power of Consciousness

Ethical dimensions of the process, as well as the content of the learning experience, are central for reaching heightened awareness. A portion of each gathering, usually toward the end, is devoted to a closing "ritual" that includes criticism, where everyone reflects on the process of the gathering, what it meant, and ways in which the intended values were enacted.

Power of Diversity

Deliberate processes are planned and enacted to integrate points of view of individuals and groups whose perspectives are usually not addressed. The experiences (through writings, personal encounters, poetry, song, drama, etc.) of minority groups, of different classes, of third-world people, of women, are given a deliberate focus during the learning experience. In nursing education, nursing itself has been so long devalued as an important resource for learning, that it represents a diversity apart from the mainstream of the health care system. Thus, nursing literature, experience, stories, and ways of knowing are consciously emphasized.

Power of Responsibility

All participants assume full responsibility as the agent for her or his role in the process. The experience is planned to provide some structure that assures every participant the opportunity to assume a leadership role during the experience. "Grades" are viewed as each individual's responsibility; they are viewed as a tool to represent what the individual earns through demonstrated accomplishments. Teachers assume responsibility to demystify the processes involved in all planned activities, including provisions for evaluation and grades and other expectations imposed by the structure of the institution.

PRACTICAL SUGGESTIONS FOR USING A FEMINIST PEDAGOGY

There are many ways in which the feminist concepts of power can be enacted in a learning situation. The suggestions here are certainly not the only way; they are examples taken from my own experience. I have used the approaches described here with groups of 6 to 40 students. The size of the groups in which the process has been most successful is about 20. Traditional pedagogies do not provide a means for everyone present to fully participate, and the shift that makes this possible begins to be most apparent in this size group.

In order to demystify all elements of the experience, I have used the course syllabus as a means of providing detailed information about the pedagogical premises and methods, as well as guidelines for the gatherings that are appropriate to the course content. I have included the structure of the curriculum: course description, objectives, and listings of texts. I have used *Peace & Power: A Handbook of Feminist Process* (Wheeler & Chinn, 1984, 1989) as a reading the first week after the group convenes as a means of introducing everyone to the group process that we will use.

The syllabus contains four major elements: philosophy of the course design, a description of the learning activities that are planned as a structure from which we can work, the suggested provisions for how each participant can earn a grade that demonstrates her or his competence, and a working outline from which the group can plan each gathering. The following sections provide examples taken from the syllabus of a first semester graduate course on nursing theory development.

EXAMPLE OF THE "PHILOSOPHY OF THE COURSE DESIGN"

The activities and interactions in this course are planned to enact the philosophy of the School of Nursing, and the philosophic basis upon which nursing theory is developed.

The emphasis is on:

- Creativity
- Humanistic care
- The autonomy and unique individuality of each participant
- The growth and development of all participants.

All participants have different and unique experiences and talents; all are valued equally. In order for the ideal of equal participation and valuing to be actualized, all participants assume full responsibility and accountability. It is the responsibility of all participants to actively value their own, and each other participant's critical thought, experiences, knowledge, and talents.

The faculty role in this experience is based on the desire to eliminate the unequal power relationships that exist within current institutionalized educational settings. The faculty is a participant and a learner along with all other participants, not the expert, judge, or "guru." The faculty enters with experience and background in relation to the focus of the course, and is responsible for preparing materials that can be used as a starting point for learning and development, providing resources for planning each discussion with the co-conveners, and for providing feedback and constructive criticism for all activities designed to demonstrate competence in relation to learning.

The faculty is obligated to provide evidence of each individual's completion of the learning objectives in the form of a grade. However, the grade for the course is earned, not given. The faculty participates with each individual in assessing work that demonstrates the grade that is earned.

EXAMPLE OF "LEARNING ACTIVITIES"

1. *Discussion Convening:* At least once each participant will work with another participant to convene the gathering. This requires in-depth reading of all the planned readings for the gathering, and meeting with faculty and/or co-convener(s) before the gathering to plan the agenda. Individuals volunteer for convening responsibilities at least one week in advance. Convening provides the opportunity to practice leadership in a safe environment, where group feedback and support can be provided.
2. *Reading and Participation in Discussion:* For each gathering there are planned readings; these and any other readings you select provide a basis for active discussion. Discussions also draw on personal experiences, so your personal journal (described below) will be important to help you reflect on the meaning of this experience.

   There are several short stories on reserve in the library that are planned for reading within the first four weeks of the semester. The purposes of the short stories are to: 1) provide a common "clinical experience" for discussion practice implications of theoretical ideas, 2) provide insight and inspiration in creative expression, and 3) provide experience related to the esthetic pattern of knowing in nursing.

Being *Present* (in mind, body, and spirit) is important both for individual learning and for the development of the group as a whole. During check-in, each participant connects with the group and uses this sharing to help everyone integrate individual needs and agendas for the gathering. If an individual must be absent, leave early, or otherwise interrupt the discussion, that individual lets *everyone* in the group know in advance so all can anticipate and plan for the shift in group dynamics.

Each discussion will conclude with appreciation, criticism, and affirmation. During this time each person reflects on the process of the gathering, the extent to which the group process facilitated individual and group development, and explores suggestions for moving ahead.

3. *Personal Journal:* All participants keep a personal journal or diary throughout the semester. The journal provides a record of your personal growth and development, and can serve as the basis for other learning activities such as group discussions or writing. The journal is not shared, except in rare instances. The central purpose of the journal is to explore avenues of personal knowing in nursing.

4. *Scholarly Writing:* A scholarly paper related to the learning objectives of the course is planned as the primary avenue for demonstrating your accomplishments. The primary purpose of the writing is to explore the potential for development of nursing knowledge. At least two drafts of the writing will be shared. One copy of each draft is shared with faculty and one copy with another participant. Reviewers provide constructive criticism in the interest of helping you develop your ideas. A suggested schedule for assuring completion of the writing during the semester is included in the detailed topical outline for the semester.

5. *Critique of Colleague's Writing:* Each participant will review a colleague's first draft of the written work and write a brief summary of suggestions and comments. These will be shared with the author to use as needed; a copy of the review will be provided for the faculty, to document your participation in this activity, and for faculty feedback to help develop this skill.

EXAMPLE OF "GRADING" PROPOSAL

Grading: All participants earn a grade of "B" on completion of the following:

- *Co-convenes* group discussions as needed to provide leadership for all the gatherings. Each participant will co-convene at least once; if the group is small, additional responsibilities for co-convening will be mutually agreed upon by the group. The quality of convening will be reflected in the criticism/self-criticism portion of the discussion; the grade is not affected.

- *Participates actively in discussion* during each gathering, with no more than 3 absences during the semester, unless negotiated differently with the entire group.
- *Provides written criticism* of a colleague's early draft(s) of written work. Copies of an adapted ANS review form are provided to facilitate developing skills of constructive criticism. The review is shared with the author of the paper, and with the faculty as evidence of completion and competence in written criticism. Reviews are not "graded," nor will they affect the grade of the author of the written work that is reviewed.
- *Prepares a scholarly essay* that is shared with faculty and with another participant in the group in draft and final forms. Every reviewer provides constructive criticism of the work-in-progress to aid the author in developing the essay. The faculty is responsible to assess the work in relation to the grade, and will discuss with the author any concerns related to the grade the individual is earning. The criteria on which a grade of "B" is based are provided on the adapted *Advances in Nursing Science* review form as follows:

  I. Consistency with the course objectives.

  II. Concise, logical ordering of ideas; readability.

  III. Sound argument and defense of original ideas.

  IV. Accuracy of content.

  V. Appropriate use of methods of scholarly investigation.

  VI. Adequacy of documentation.

"A" Grade: An "A" grade is earned by demonstrating excellence. An "A" grade is earned by individuals who:

- Demonstrate competence in all planned learning activities.
- Participate actively in all gatherings, with no more than one absence during the semester.
- Share an enrichment project with the group that is contracted with the group as a whole. The group is responsible to agree that the project is related to our mutual goals and that it will provide enrichment for the individual and for the group.

"C" Grade or lower: The processes of the course are designed to provide maximum opportunity for early, open feedback; discussion; and negotiation along the way to assure that each participant earns the grade that is sought. A grade of "C" or lower will be recorded if these processes are not successful.

Incomplete grade: Incompletes will not be used for this course; if you begin to have problems in completing the learning activities, you are urged to consult with faculty as early as possible, and to withdraw from the course.

EXAMPLE OF DETAILED "TOPICAL OUTLINE"

The following are extracts from a complete topical outline. These extracts illustrate the planning for a gradual development of writing skills and learning the skills of providing constructive critique of a colleague's writing. The suggested readings illustrate the integration of a diversity of "voices" and avenues for introducing a perspective based on women's experiences of the world.

WEEK #2: **DEVELOPMENT OF KNOWLEDGE** (SEPTEMBER 19)

(Course Objectives: 1.1, 1.2, 1.3)

Conveners: ______________________________

Readings:

Phillips, D. C. (1987). *Philosophy, science and social inquiry* (Part A: Expositions: Recent philosophical developments, pp. 2–45). New York: Pergamon.

Spender, Dale. (1982). *Invisible women: The schooling scandal* (Introduction, Chapters 1 & 2, pp. 1–38). London: Writers and Readers Publishing Cooperative.

Wheeler, Charlene Eldridge & Chinn, Peggy L. (1985). *Peace and Power: A Handbook of Feminist Process.* Buffalo: Margaretdaughters, Inc.

Woolf, Virginia. (1979). Women and fiction. In M. Barrett (Ed.), *Virginia Woolf: Women and writing* (pp. 43–52). New York: Harcourt Brace Jovanovich. (Reprinted from *The Forum,* 1929).

Selected Short Stories. The stories that are on reserve include:

Browne, Susan E.: "Infusing Blues." True story of a nurse with diabetes and her struggle in gaining control. (biographical)

Finger, Annie: "Like the Hully Gully but Not So Slow." True story of a teenager with physical disability and her conflicts with her family. (biographical)

Geller, Ruth: "The Island." Story of a nurse dealing with the stress of her work/personal life. (fiction)

Geller, Ruth: "The Woman with My Eyes." Story involving a patient from Buffalo Psych Center and a worker in the experimental laboratory. (fiction)

Gilman, Charlotte Perkins: "The Yellow Wallpaper." Story of postpartum depression. (partly autobiographical, partly fiction)

LeGuin, Ursula K.: "Mazes." Story involving scientific experimentation. (fiction)

O'Connor, Flannery: "The Geranium." Story of an old man's day-today survival. (fiction)

Olsen, Tillie: "I Stand Here Ironing." Story involving a mother's reflections on raising her troubled daughter. (fiction)

Rose, Susan: "Pictures from a Family Album." Story told in the voice of an abused child. (? fiction)

Learning Activities:

Begin personal journal.

Suggestion: Reflect on the meaning of the readings to you, write about experiences and events that remind you of readings this week.

WEEK #3: PHILOSOPHY AND HISTORY OF NURSING SCIENCE (SEPTEMBER 26)

(Course Objectives 3.1, 3.3)

Conveners: ______________________________

Readings:

Carper, Barbara. (1987, October). Fundamental patterns of knowing in nursing. *Advances in Nursing Science, 1*(1), 13–23.

Chinn, Peggy L. & Jacobs, Maeona Kramer. (1987). *Theory and nursing: A systematic approach* (2nd ed.) (Chapters 1 and 2, pp. 1–62). St. Louis: Mosby.

Silva, Mary C. & Rothbart, Daniel (1984, January). An analysis of changing trends in philosophies of science on nursing theory development and testing. *Advances in Nursing Science, 6*(2), 1–13. (See also Letter to the Editor in *ANS 9*(2), January 1987.)

Learning Activities:

Continue work on personal journal.
Begin exploring topics for scholarly essay.

Suggestion: Make a list of "burning questions" about nursing and your specialty area of practice, and begin discussing them with your colleagues.

WEEK #4: WHAT IS THEORY AND WHY DOES IT EXIST? (OCTOBER 3)

(Course objectives 1.1, 2.1)

Conveners: ______________________________

Readings:

Bunch, Charlotte (1987). Not by degrees: Feminist theory and education. In C. Bunch (Ed.), *Passionate politics: Feminist theory in action,* (pp. 240–253) New York: St. Martin's Press.

Chinn, Peggy L. & Jacobs, Maeona K. (1987). *Theory and nursing: A systematic approach* (2nd ed.) (Chapter 3, pp. 64–85). St. Louis: Mosby.

Kindilien, Carlin. (1982). *Basic writing skills* (Part Four: A Writing Procedure, pp. 71–97). New York: Arco.

Meleis, Afaf I. (1985). *Theoretical nursing: Development and progress* (Chapter 5, pp. 79–106). Philadelphia: Lippincott.

Stember, Marilyn (1986). Model building as a strategy for theory development. In P. L. Chinn (Ed.), *Nursing research methodology: Issues and implementation* (pp. 103–119). Rockville, MD: Aspen Publishers.

Learning Activities:

Continue work on personal journal.
Work on Stage I from Kindilien.

Suggestion: Select one of your "burning questions" and try to frame a main sentence around this question.

WEEK #7: **EVALUATION OF THEORY** (OCTOBER 24)

(Course Objectives 1.1, 1.6, 4.1, 4.2, 4.3, 4.4)

Conveners: ____________________

Readings:

Chinn, Peggy L. & Jacobs, Maeona K. (1987). *Theory and nursing: A systematic approach* (2nd ed.) (Chapter 6, pp. 134–148). St. Louis: Mosby.
Ramos, Mary Carol. (1987). Adopting an evolutionary lens: An optimistic approach to discovering strength in nursing. *Advances in Nursing Science, 10*(1), 19–26.

Learning Activities:

Continue work on personal journal.
Complete Kindilien's Stage 3.

Suggestion: Kindilien's suggestions are wonderful! Set aside about 3 hours to sit down and do it. Work with a word processor if possible; write no more than about 4 to 5 pages at this stage. Read what you have written to get a general idea of immediate impressions you want to tend to now, but then let it rest and don't work with it any more.

SHARE DRAFT OF YOUR SCHOLARLY WRITING at the October 24 gathering. Be sure to bring 2 copies of your work; one for faculty and one for another participant.

WEEK #8: **THEORY, PRACTICE, AND RESEARCH LINKS** (OCTOBER 31)

(Course objectives 1.4, 1.5, 1.6, 2.1, 3.1, 3.2, 4)

Conveners: ____________________

Readings:

Benner, Patricia & Tanner, Christine. (1987, January). How expert nurses use intuition. *American Journal of Nursing, 87*(1), 23–31.
Chinn, Peggy L. & Jacobs, Maeona K. (1987). *Theory and nursing: A systematic approach* (2nd ed.) (Chapters 7 & 8, pp. 150–180). St. Louis: Mosby.
Fawcett, Jacquelyn. (1979, October). The relationship between theory and research: A double-helix. *Advances in Nursing Science, 1*(1), 49–62.
Quinn, Janet F. (1984, January). Therapeutic touch as energy exchange. *Advances in Nursing Science, 6*(2), 42–49.

Learning Activities:

Continue work on personal journal.
Complete your critique of your colleague's scholarly writing. Use the adapted *ANS* review form.

Suggestion: Be constructive. Point out things about the writing that need improvement and offer suggestions for making the changes needed. Don't worry about whether you are "correct"—simply share your impressions with the author. Remember that this is not meant to be a finished product; your comments will help the author to refine the writing. Comment on both the content of the writing and the presentation or style.

SHARE YOUR REVIEW WITH THE AUTHOR AND RETURN THE DRAFT TO THE AUTHOR at the October 31 gathering.

REFERENCES

Daly, M., & Caputi, J. (1987). *Websters' first new intergalactic wickedary of the English language.* Boston: Beacon Press.

Harding, S. (1987). *Feminism and methodology: Social science issues.* Bloomington: Indiana University Press.

Spender, D. (1982). *Invisible women: The schooling scandal.* London: Writers and Readers Publishing Cooperative.

Weiler, K. (1988). *Women teaching for change: Gender, class & power.* South Hadley, MA: Bergin & Garvey.

Wheeler, C. E. & Chinn, P. L. (1984). *Peace and power: A handbook of feminist process.* Buffalo, NY: Margaretdaughters.

Wheeler, C. E., & Chinn, P. L. (1989). *Peace and power: A handbook of feminist process* (2nd ed.). New York: National League for Nursing.

BIBLIOGRAPHY

Allen, D. (1985, Summer). Nursing research and social control: Alternative models of science that emphasize understanding and emancipation. *Image, 17*(2), 58–64.

Anderson, J. M. (1985, October). Perspectives on the health of immigrant women: A feminist analysis. *Advances in Nursing Science, 8*(1), 61–76.

Andolsen, B. H., Gudorf, C. E., & Pellauer, M. D. (Eds.). (1985). *Women's consciousness, women's conscience: A reader in feminist ethics.* New York: Harper & Row.

Bleier, R. (Ed.). (1986). *Feminist approaches to science.* New York: Pergamon Press.

Bunch, C. (1987). *Passionate politics: Feminist theory in action.* New York: St. Martin's Press.

Charleston Faculty Practice Conference Group. (1986, January). Nursing faculty collaboration viewed through feminist process. *Advances in Nursing Science, 8*(2), 29–38.

Chinn, P. L., & Wheeler, C. E. (1985, March/April). Feminism and nursing. *Nursing Outlook, 33*(2), 74–77.

Christian, B. (1988, Spring). The race for theory. *Feminist Studies, 14*(1), 67–79.

Crowley, M. A. (1989, April). Feminist pedagogy: Nurturing the ethical ideal. *Advances in Nursing Science, 11*(3).

Daly, M. (1978). *Gyn/Ecology: The metaethics of radical feminism.* Boston: Beacon Press.

Daly, M., & Caputi, J. (1987). *Websters' first new intergalactic wickedary of the English language.* Boston: Beacon Press.

Davis, A. Y. (1981). *Women, race & class.* New York: Random House.

Donovan, J. (1985). *Feminist theory: The intellectual traditions of American feminism.* New York: Ungar.

Ecker, G. (Ed.). (1986). *Feminist aesthetics.* Boston: Beacon Press.

Freire, P. (1970). *Pedagogy of the oppressed.* New York: The Seabury Press.

Frye, M. (1983). *The politics of reality: Essays in feminist theory.* Trumansburg, NY: The Crossing Press.

Greene, G. & Kahn, C. (Eds.). (1985). *Making a difference: Feminist literary criticism.* New York: Methuen.

Harding, S. (1986). *The science question in feminism.* Ithaca: Cornell University Press.

Harding, S. (Ed.). (1987). *Feminism and methodology: Social science issues.* Bloomington: Indiana University Press.

Heide, W. S. (1985). *Feminism for the health of it.* Buffalo, NY: Margaretdaughters.

Hooks, B. (1981). *Ain't I a woman: Black women and feminism.* Boston: South End Press.

Hooks, B. (1984). *Feminist theory: From margin to center.* Boston: South End Press.

Jagger, A. M., & Rothenberg, P. S. (1984). *Feminist frameworks: Alternative theoretical accounts of the relations between women and men* (2nd ed.). New York: McGraw-Hill.

Keller, E. F. (1985). *Reflections on gender and science.* New Haven: Yale University Press.

Leavitt, J. W., & Gordon, L. (1988, Autumn). A decade of feminist critiques in the natural science: An address by Ruth Bleier. *Signs: Journal of Women in Culture and Society, 14*(1), 182–195.

MacPherson, K. I. (1983, January). Feminist methods: A new paradigm for nursing research. *Advances in Nursing Science, 5*(2), 17–25.

MacPherson, K. I. (1985, July). Osteoporosis and menopause: A feminist analysis of the social construction of a syndrome. *Advances in Nursing Science, 7*(4), 11–22.

MacPherson, K. I. (1986). *Feminist praxis in the making: The menopause collective.* Doctoral dissertation, Boston: Brandeis University.

Moraga, C., & Anzaldua, G. (Eds.). (1981). *This bridge called my back: Writings by radical women of color.* New York: Kitchen Table Press.

Newton, J., & Rosenfelt, D. (Eds.). (1985). *Feminist criticism and social change: Sex, class and race in literature and culture.* New York: Methuen.

Raymond, J. G. (1986). *A passion for friends: Toward a philosophy of female affection.* Boston: Beacon Press.

Reinharz, S., & Davidman, L. (1988). *Social science methods, feminist voices: Readings and interpretations.* New York: Pergamon Books.

Roberts, H. (Ed.). (1981). *Doing feminist research.* Boston: Routledge & Kegan Paul.

Rosser, S. V. (1986). *Teaching science and health from a feminist perspective: A practical guide.* New York: Pergamon Press.

Rothschild, J. (Ed.). (1983). *Machina ex dea: Feminist perspectives on technology.* New York: Pergamon Press.

Showalter, E. (Ed.). (1985). *The new feminist criticism: Essays on women, literature, and theory.* New York: Pantheon.

Spender, D. (1982a). *Invisible women: The schooling scandal.* London: Writers and Readers Publishing Cooperative.

Spender, D. (1982b). *Women of ideas and what men have done to them: From Aphra Behn to Adrienne Rich.* Boston: Routledge & Kegan Paul.

Stanley, L., & Wise, S. (1983). *Breaking out: Feminist consciousness and feminist research.* Boston: Routledge & Kegan Paul.

Thompson, J. L. (1987, October). Critical scholarship: The critique of domination in nursing. *Advances in Nursing Science, 10*(1), 27–38.

Walker, A. (1983). *In search of our mothers' gardens: Womanist prose.* New York: Harcourt Brace Jovanovich.

Weiler, K. (1988). *Women teaching for change: Gender, class & power.* South Hadley, MA: Bergin & Garvey.

Wheeler, C. E., & Chinn, P. L. (1984). *Peace and power: A handbook of feminist process.* Buffalo, NY: Margaretdaughters.

Wheeler, C. E., & Chinn, P. L. (1989). *Peace and power: A handbook of feminist process* (2nd ed.). New York: National League for Nursing.

3

The Nursing Curriculum: Lived Experiences of Students

Nancy L. Diekelmann, PhD, RN, FAAN

> The world created by developing and implementing a nursing curriculum is a world inhabited by people. It is an actively lived-in world and a meaning world. In every revolution, there occurs times that require moments of free play and intellectual legroom. When nurse educators become learners and explore the question of what it means to be a nursing student, the opportunity for free play unfolds. New approaches that ground nursing education in the lived-experiences of students emerge. We live the revolution through the continual rebirth of our struggle to understand. (Diekelmann, 1986)

As we struggle to understand both our practice of teaching in nursing and the nature of nursing education as teaching and learning, hermeneutic inquiry can help us uncover new understandings. Hermeneutics is not an end in itself, but a way of entering into the horizonal understanding of the nature of teaching and learning in nursing. Hermeneutic inquiry is constitutive of education that both situates learning and empowers students and teachers as they struggle together to understand. It can also be a research method to analyze the voices of students, teachers, clinicians, and patients, uncovering hidden meanings and relationships.

Dialogue as hermeneutic inquiry can illuminate the "Being-in" phenomenon of groups. Being-in-the-world (Heidegger, 1962) as inhabiting,

---

I am indebted to Patricia Benner for her seminal nursing studies, which have introduced Heideggerian hermeneutical approaches into the discipline of nursing. I also extend my gratitude to Louise Shores, who initiated the returning registered nurse study that I have had the privilege to extend. Lastly, I thank all the students who have shared their experiences with me, affording me a privileged view of their world.

is the how of the kind of being we are. Being-in is the language (Heidegger, 1971a), embodied understandings (Merleau-Ponty, 1962) and practices that are enlightening for us to uncover and understand.

I will first present my hermeneutic studies of the lived experiences of students in all levels and types of nursing programs (Diekelmann, 1988). A relational theme, **Learning as Evaluation,** will be described, followed by the **Constitutive Pattern: Being in Practice—Returning to School** that emerged from my interviews of returning registered nurses. The second part of the chapter will be a reconceptualization of the nursing **Curriculum as Dialogue and Meaning,** focusing on the teacher-as-learner and the curriculum-as-dialogue. The chapter will conclude with a discussion of issues for educators to be in dialogue about as we struggle to understand more about the nature of our teaching/learning and practical activity.

LEARNING AS EVALUATION

Learning as Evaluation is a relational theme that emerged across the hermeneutical interviews of diploma, associate degree, baccalaureate, and graduate students. Voice after voice spoke of their lived experiences of being evaluated, preparing for, or coping with evaluation. In a sister hermeneutic study of teachers in nursing, I was impressed by the large number of instances where teachers described grading care plans, writing anecdotal notes, writing test items, and grading papers. Teachers reported that they spent "enormous" amounts of time on these activities.

A commitment to teaching as evaluation reflects behavioral education. Learning as a change in behavior and evaluation as evidence of it are the hallmarks of behavioral approaches. The paradox of this commitment to teaching as evaluation—by both students and teachers—is reflected in the following analogy.

The American hemisphere contains over a million species of insects, less than 1 percent are pests; defined as being destructive of or dangerous to plants and animals. Paradoxically when we think of insects, we think of the one percent: mosquitoes, bees, or others, ignoring the other 99 percent. This gives us an inaccurate understanding of the nature of the insect world.

On a daily basis we are taught, and we learn things that are never formally evaluated, yet we have come to equate the teaching we do with formal evaluation. I will argue that while formal evaluation is a part of teaching and learning it constitutes the very smallest part of the basis of what we do.

As a part of the revolution, we need to discuss the meaning of evaluation among ourselves and our students. We need to examine the assumption that if learning has not been evaluated, we cannot know or prove that it has occurred. The experience of teachers and students negates this assumption. As we live the paradox of learning as evaluation, we can examine whether we want to continue spending so much of our time on formal evaluation. Evaluation many only prove to ourselves and our students what we often already know. Perhaps understanding the students' lived experiences and the meanings of evaluation will help us transform evaluation as a part of practice in teaching nursing.

Learning as Evaluation: Adversarialism in Action

Evaluation was frequently experienced as adversarial by all types of students from diploma to graduate. Often students described feelings of frustration and anger.

> I never know what this teacher wants. I'm serious! I trust someone at first, you know until I learn better. . . . I don't listen to what other students have to say about teachers I get. . . . I give them a chance—that's only fair. But this teacher, the one in charge of the course, said, "I won't test you on the first two chapters." Well, sure enough on the exam, she did. And when we complained in class, she said, "Well, it's only 5 points, and anyway, you should know it, as it was covered in class. . . ." I just can't trust her now at all.

Occasionally both students and teachers were interviewed regarding a similar event. The complexity of evaluating learning, in this instance writing exams, emerges in this teacher's description of writing this exam.

> I had 12 lectures to cover in this unit exam and 9 different people who presented the content . . . and each gave me questions. Some were well written, but I thought too hard. Others were over points that were unimportant. . . . and of course, a full professor who gave 2 lectures turned in this long, incredibly difficult question. Her lecture was at odds with the chapter in the book, and she contradicted herself several times in class. I was up until 1 A.M. writing this darn thing so the secretary could get it typed and duplicated . . . and I knew I would have to talk to everyone about all the things I had done with their questions, and there was no time to meet again to discuss the exam. I really don't have time to run around to all of them and call them and wait for them to call me back. . . . Writing exams, especially new ones, is something I hate! Then the students are all over you. You said this and you said that. It gets to a point with 80-some students, I can't remember what I said sometimes. They drive you nuts, always wanting to know what's going to be on the test. I get asked that so many times and places—even in the bathroom. . . . If students would spend as much time on learning as they would on trying to figure out what not to study, they'd do just fine. . . . When I go into class to go over the exams, I feel like I'm going into battle!

In his analysis of adversarialism in America, William May (1988) compares professionalism, that is the structural relationships of the client and the professional, to the relationship of the citizen to the Lockean state—a contractarian and adversarial outlook which, he argues, "dominates the American scene" (p. 187). This comparison, using the profession of teaching, posits that:

1. The relationship would be characterized by the teacher owning original authority to the threat of a negative.
2. Students are relatively passive beneficiaries of powers exercised by others.
3. Students are largely active only at the entry and exit into the school or course.
4. The contract between the teacher and the student is one that encourages transactional rather than transformational understanding of the nature of the exchange.

Briefly, teaching as evaluation begins to unveil how the nature of teaching as evaluation and the practices shared with and among teachers and students have become adversarial. Teachers in many of the interviews emerged as the gatekeepers of the profession of nursing. Embedded within this theme is the negative assumption that without teachers evaluating, the public would have unsafe nurses caring for them. Our profession has always feared that without evaluation as part of nursing instruction, the public might be at the mercy of unqualified practitioners. While the intent may be worthy, the means to achieve this—such as scores on examinations—are indeed fraught with difficulties that belie the intent.

The behavioral model of nursing education encourages a teacher-centered relationship (Giroux, 1988a). In this model teachers have both the right and the responsibility for evaluation (Feinburg, 1983; Giroux, 1988b). Students are included in the planning, managing, and evaluating of the experiences, but if there is conflict over a test item, the teacher has the final power and authority. Students are often asked for input, but usually at the beginning and end of a course rather than on a ongoing, day-to-day basis.

Finally, the nature of what students and teachers do together is unfortunately transactional rather than transformative as it could be. The intent of the teacher is focused on creating change in the intellectual and technical skills that are mediated through transactions between and among teachers and students. The intent is not to transform the teachers' understanding of what it means to care for certain patients—rather it is to teach care of these certain patients to nursing students. The theme of education as evaluation is fruitful to consider from the perspective of adversarialism.

There were other meanings than adversarialism embedded in students' accounts of learning taking the form of evaluation. As Cynthia's story unfolds, her frustration over a required presentation emerges.

> I—we—had to talk, give a presentation on something within the nursing field or the health medical field, and I talked about the medically indigent, and in my critique she couldn't understand what that had to do with the health field, and just went on to say that she really didn't understand what my point was of speaking on the medically indigent, and *I had to proceed to tell her* that it was an ever-growing problem, especially now when people, if people don't have insurance, don't have access to the medical services, then people are sicker, people aren't seeking out the care they need. And she just, I don't know, we kind of went around and around about why I thought that was important and why I thought that had to do with something in the medical field. I don't know, I had a hard time with her. As a person, I got along with her. As an instructor, *I didn't know what her motives were.*

Ironically this example reflects the very solution to transforming education. According to Shor (1986):

> Students will resist any process that disempowers them. Unequal, disabling education is symbolic violence against them, which they answer with their own skills of resistance—silence, disruption, nonperformance, cheating, lateness, absence, vandalism, etc. Very familiar school routines produce this alienation: teacher-talk, passive instruction in preset materials, punitive testing . . . , . . . denial of themes and other subjects important to them, the exclusion of student co-participation in curriculum design and governance. . . . (p. 183)

The self-directed school can hope to reverse these conditions only with an empowering, critical pedagogy. We need to consider how we can achieve reconciliation between students and ourselves to reduce hostility and to foster community instead of alienation. Perhaps many nursing students, on all levels, are on strike.

> Goodlad observed 1000 classrooms over an eight-year period and reported: Teachers appear to teach within a very limited repertoire of pedagogical alternatives, emphasizing their own talk. This customary pedagogy places the teacher in control. Few activities call for or even permit active student planning. Students listen, they respond when called on to do so. They read and chose from alternative responses in quizzes. But they rarely plan or initiate anything. (Shor, 1986, p. 187)

But empowering pedagogies are constantly under regressive pressure from the way of past traditions (Apple, 1986; Greene, 1988; Weiler, 1988). The old script of teacher-talk and student-silence is a formidable presence that needs constant practice for reversal. We need to conduct research on the practice of teaching to see how teachers are able to resist this regressive pressure on a day-to-day basis. Not only do we need to explore dilemmas teachers confront but also the transformations that occur. It is important to make excellence visible in the practice of teaching in order to have a future of possibilities.

As teachers we need to find ways to reconcile and empower students in the curriculum. Many students are angry and feeling controlled and manipulated, although this not the intent of the faculty. It is timely to explore how the "factory model" (Kliebard, 1977) of behavioral education has encouraged this and discouraged many teachers from considering other alternatives that empower and engage students in their own learning. Rather than seeking new "approaches" or curricular models, we should explore new ways of being for ourselves, with each other, our students, and our clinical colleagues. Hermeneutic inquiry and dialogue are two hopeful possibilities. As we explore our lived experience and the phenomenon of language as we are in the world, new approaches will emerge that illuminate how we can be in our schools. This concern with *how* we are in the world can occur today. It is a struggle we all experience.

Experience and Learning as Evaluation—Returning Registered Nurses

Learning as Evaluation was an issue for returning registered nurse students. They often spoke of struggling to reconcile their own views and understanding of their personal knowledge and skills as inconsistent with the grades or evaluations they received from their teachers. Of particular concern to many were all forms of written examinations. One student, Ted, explains his struggle to understand why he is so unsuccessful with exams in a nursing course he is taking:

> I understand that tests in a baccalaureate program are not of the same type as AD [Associate Degree]. . . . I realize these tests are not to prepare me for Boards, like I always thought my AD courses did. . . . In this course I'm in now, the *questions are written different that what I've experienced.* . . . I know the information, but I can't answer those questions. And it's like, I'm not sure what the questions are asking. *There's always that little question mark?* I'm somehow different when I take tests—or *how* a test is different for me now that I've practiced.

This theme, Learning as Evaluation points toward the paradox of evaluation in which teachers seek to teach rules to students but want them eventually to recognize when and how to modify or not use them. Students with clinical experience have learned to read situations: they feel hampered when confined to a written description which does not allow them an opportunity to see, hear, and/or speak in the situation as an integral part of judgment-making. Studies show that nurses' engagement in the total situation is crucial to making clinical judgments (Benner, 1984; Benner & Tanner, 1987; Benner & Wrubel, 1989; Tanner, Padrick, Westfall, & Puzier, 1987).

Teachers write examinations for students to test the acontextual rules they have been given in class, which assumes that students have not had experiences that dictate that these rules be transformed. Students encounter difficulty because they understand, and find most meaningful, rules in their transformed states. An important goal in teaching clinical judgment-making is unveiling the irony inherent in this seeming conflict.

Teachers describe that ideally they want students to know not merely these basic rules, but also when to apply and when to alter them. Yet they are faced with the practical difficulty of classes requiring machine-graded test items and forms of evaluation that are based on making simple causal relationships to achieve the correct answer. Significant about the struggle of many students with clinical experience was their inability to associate their difficulty in taking the examination with the role experience played on their ability to select the correct answer. They attributed their difficulty either to a poorly written examination, inability to take these kinds of exams, or their personal abilities. Many students were unable to associate their difficulty in exams with their experiences. Only a few were aware that their experience had influenced their judgment. Most students seemed only marginally aware that perhaps practice has influenced the way they read situations, making strictly written accounts difficult for them. There was little awareness that their understanding of the causal relationships required of the exams had been transformed through their practical experience.

We need to struggle to develop examinations that allow for the recognition of transformative understandings. The influence of our current kinds of evaluation needs to be analyzed. For example, do students learn as nurses how to capitulate to the teacher as an authority figure? Faced with situations of conflict between their experiential and intuitive understandings and the theoretical understandings demanded by the test, do they learn diminished respect for practical knowledge? More fundamentally, we need to explore how and in what ways practice experiences have transformed how these students learn, think, and write. In this way, teachers can engage in more meaningful dialogues with these experienced students.

Constitutive Pattern: Being in Practice—Returning to School

For many students, returning to school was a story of great personal sacrifices and turmoil. Some described divorces, impending or emerging; others, severe financial constraints or family responsibilities.

Ivy was faced with a divorce, twin four-year-olds and a full-time job. She described her former husband's resistance to her returning to school. Tuition was a problem, and she had to take out loans. "Being bound and determined" to complete her degree, she told of having to convince her former husband that:

> I will have a better job and I'll have, you know, make better money, *whether any of that is true or not.* He's convinced that after I get out of school, I'll be more marketable, which I don't really know is true. He frankly doesn't want me to be in school and have my time taken away from him, our children, and keeping house. He thinks college is stupid.

Returning to school for Ivy was both a hardship and a transforming experience. She examines her oppression and the relationship she had had with her husband in the context of returning to school for her baccalaureate degree.

She was very frank in her explanations of how she coped with a full-time job, her family, and school. Describing that she often got behind but worked well under pressure, Ivy told of an incident in which she had a paper due.

> It was during the winter, and the warmest and quietest place was, well it was quiet, it had to be because it was late at night and I didn't want to disturb my husband. I was cold too, my husband turned the heat down and the warmest place was in our bathroom. *So the stool was my writing desk, and I was on the floor, I sat on the floor, and wrote for hours, using the toilet stool as my desk.* And for some reason, that worked well. It was, you know, I guess because *I knew I had a deadline to meet, and that's just what I had to do.* That's why sometimes if a paper is late and my teacher penalizes me or acts like I did it on purpose, she just doesn't understand. I'd love to get my papers done on time. Sometimes I just can't. . . . that's why I say, studying's real difficult for me, just finding out the time, and then sitting there, buckling down to do it, because *swimming* in my head, if I don't get rid of all those thoughts, it's: "What am I going to do at work the next day?" You know, so and so called me, she wants this favor done. I've got a husband and kids, you know, "What am I ever going to feed them? Am I ever going grocery shopping?"

Many students explained how they came to understand more about nursing, what nursing was, and what it meant to them. They began to realize that they are forever different kinds of learners because they have been in practice. Some students even told of being disappointed that they could no longer study and learn nursing the way they did it "the first time." Nursing practice and caring, for many of the returning registered nurse students, both informed and shaped their lives as students. The practice of nursing had deep meanings for their lives. In fact, a grounding in practice was so meaningful for them that many clung to their part-time practices, even when they didn't need the money or could have taken respite without losing their skills.

For many of these returning students, it was in practice that they were able to discuss the new meanings that were emerging from their schooling. Some talked of weekly sharing with the nurses on their unit about what had been covered in class; others talked about the memorable times when something they had heard or read clicked. This constant dialogue about their practical experiences is both problematic and empowering for them. At times when they have the wrong answer because they considered a variable that was not explicit on the test, it was problematic. But when the nature of practice enhanced their ability to make intelligible the information they had received in class or gave them learning skills they needed to complete assignments, it was enabling and empowering. This student talked about how her practice experiences enabled her:

> I have learned how to study and figure things out. I am a really good listener, because on our unit—neuro—things change so fast there is not time to read and keep up. That would be impossible. You just have to catch what you can as the docs or the CNS tell you or someone else something. And because we do so much diagnostic work, I've learned to listen very, very, very closely—oh so closely to patients. I listen with my ears, my eyes, my heart, and my soul! . . . But also I know how to use the library and scan things for what is most important in an article. We are always having something on the unit that we haven't seen before, and one of us has to go look things up in the library. So I guess you might say that as a part of my job, just being a neuro nurse, I'm used to studying.

Embedded in many accounts of experiences by returning registered nurses was an understanding of the meaning of being in practice *as* one returns to school. The next student first discussed her "not wanting to enter school with my back up."

> I know that most RNs don't want to be made to repeat a lot of stuff, and they feel their nursing skills and knowledge is not respected by teachers . . . Well, I knew all that, but I didn't want to go in with being negative. So I said to myself, so what if there is a little repetition, you can always learn something—or you know, learn on your own. Well, that lasted about three weeks . . . ! After two semesters, I was really discouraged. All I felt like I was doing was spending x amount of money and x amount of time, and I was going to end up with a piece of paper that says I can do what I can already do. I felt like, well, if they want me to get my degree at this hospital, I will. I will play the game, and I'll get my piece of paper.

Later this student told of taking a course where she met a teacher who, she said, "really got us thinking."

> She didn't know a whole lot clinically, but she would ask you questions, and you could see that she was really interested in how *you* were thinking. And she wanted you to get excited about your own questions. . . . I thought that was strange—teacher wanting to know what I didn't know and then giving me course credit for getting going on some answers. . . . You know, not us studying what she thought was important, but us—the students. It was the best med-surg course I ever had. And the baccalaureate students, who hadn't cared for patients but who all had interests in some kind of care were really turned on too. [This experience] really helped my attitude, because I realized that I could do what I did in that course anytime. You know, I realized my problem was not why did you come here, but how did you come here. . . . I mean I was real dense until I figured out that this happened to me in nursing too. . . . After I finally had enough experience to put in a day, I found nursing getting like a job. The work was hard. We were always short staffed, and it was tiring, boring sometimes. You got it? . . . and I found myself just going through the motions some days. Actually it scared me because one day I was feeding a lady, and I accidentally spilled some food on her, and she screamed at me—"I can't feed myself, but I'm still a person." Wow, I realized I better do something different or get out. You know that woman's comment just slapped me in the face.

This student's understanding is that it is not new information or skills or even proving that she has these that matter; rather it is the manner in which she returns. The epiphany for this student is making the link between the meaningful questions that drive her practice and the way she becomes involved in them. She sees a parallel between her experience in practice and in returning to school. It is an understanding that what matters primarily is how she comports herself in learning situations.

She described her coursework as not being meaningful and commented that learning was nothing new; expressing an alienated view of nursing education. The implications of this story are broad when we consider the increasing number of these kinds of students returning to school. We need to analyze their situations in order to better understand how to reunite returning nurses and nursing education to create a meaningful, transformative experience. Developing courses and curricula that are based in practice or are equally informed by clinicians can help to focus on bringing this transformation about. We must struggle with understanding how and in what way these kinds of experiences connect meanings for students. Hermeneutic analyses place phenomena before teachers for dialogue.

Summary

Certain assumptions about language are a part of the background for conducting hermeneutical research. According to Weber (1986):

> Language is not a neutral medium that passes freely and easily into the private property of the speaker's intentions; it is populated—overpopulated—with the intentions of others. Expropriating it, forcing it to submit to one's own intentions, is a difficult and complex process. Language is inseparable from the lived experience and the development of how people create a distinctive voice.

If we want to understand what it means to be a teacher or a student of nursing, then we must conduct research that will enable us to hear those voices. Studies grounded in hermeneutical phenomenology, first worked out by Martin Heidegger in *Being and Time* (1962), contribute to our understanding of schooling in nursing. Hermeneutical inquiry offers paths to ways of listening that will widen our understanding of the nature of teaching. Through this struggle to understand schooling in nursing, new possibilities will emerge. I am proposing a revolution that begins fundamentally within and among us.

THE CURRICULUM AS DIALOGUE AND MEANING

Heideggerian hermeneutical phenomenology offers a new way to approach nursing education that is in concert with the nature of nursing practice. In my research on the **Curriculum as Dialogue and Meaning,** I am continuing my study of the culture of nursing to understand both how nurses comport themselves and how they learn to read human comportment. Stated another way, we both constitute, or shape and are constituted or shaped by, our very existence; realization of this can be both empowering and emancipatory.

Nurses concern themselves with patterns of social behavior, patterns of actions, and adherence to social institutions, as well as with being a part of the meaning of these institutions themselves. Interpretative nursing research, in concert with the work of Paul Riceoür (1984–1986) and Donald Polkinghorne (1988), can contribute to what is described as narrative knowing. The practice of nursing is situated in an ontology of care as understanding of meaningful human action. Exciting possibilities arise when we, as researchers, wed the analyses of texts *and* actions.

As the background to discussing the **Curriculum as Dialogue and Meaning,** I will explain some of Martin Heidegger's work. His concern about our modern epoch is that we understand our human way of being as subjects with desires to be satisfied by objects which are to be controlled and used. According to Dreyfus (Magee, 1987), Heidegger later argued that we are beginning to understand everything, even ourselves, as resources to be enhanced and used efficiently. Lived experiences are lost in "enframement."

> These are all different understandings of what it is to be a thing, what it is to be a person, what it is to be an institution. Heidegger would say they are different understandings of what it is to be, and that when the understanding of what it is to be changes, *different sorts of human beings and things show up.* (Magee, 1987, p. 271)

If teachers developed hermeneutic skills—hearing rather than listening—then different sorts of human beings and things would show up for them.

What Heideggerian phenomenology offers is more than a critique of the technological understanding of being. It is also a call of concern that we are leading lives where everything is becoming as flexible as possible so as to be used as efficiently as possible. Dreyfus (Magee, 1987) describes it in this way:

> We don't seek truth any more but simply efficiency. . . . We went through a stage about a century ago when to be real or important things had to be useful for satisfying our desires. That was the subject-object stage. But now we are ourselves becoming resources in a cybernetic society where to be real is to be used as efficiently as possible. . . . We thus become part of a system which no one directs but which moves toward the total mobilization of all beings, even us, for their own welfare. Heidegger would say that the problem is there are no guidelines any more. There are no goals. Why are we concerned with using our time more and more efficiently? To what end? Just to have time to organize our lives even more efficiently? *Heidegger thinks there will soon be no meaningful differences, differences with content, any more, such as heroes and villains, or even differences like local and international, but only the more and more efficient ordering of everything, everywhere, just for the sake of more and more efficiency.* (Magee, 1987, p. 273)

We must attempt to understand why we are working so hard to organize our nursing curricula more effectively. Our view of curricula needing "organizing" is so pervasive that it constitutes for some the totality of a curriculum. That is, a curricula is the way to organize courses *into* a school.[1]

An alternative would be to consider the curriculum as a dialogue in which teachers discuss with students and clinicians the possibilities for students as they study nursing. Courses could be offered with students organizing their own "curriculum." Through dialogue with everyone concerned, we could debate our assumptions that underlie a prescribed curriculum, e.g., whether everyone must have a pediatric course or content. The meanings behind this assumption would be expressed by all; that is, teachers who feel strongly that this is an integral, necessary part of practice unique in focus and crucial to basic preparation can

[1] For a more complete analysis see: "The curriculum as tinker toy—Instrumentalism and curricular praxis" in N. Diekelmann, D. Allen & C. Tanner (in press).

debate with faculty who feel that the curriculum is currently so overloaded with information, resulting in superficial or integrated courses. These courses may not do justice to all specialty areas, so that in-depth courses would be better. Some faculty might argue for a longer period of study and more required courses or credits. Some would argue for reducing credits and changing to a twelve-month program. Clinicians could express their concerns that if students were not introduced to all areas, they might be prejudiced against certain areas. Other clinicians may prefer that students be allowed to specialize and spend enough time in clinical and coursework on one area to learn how to think as a nurse in that area. Students could discuss their concerns about not taking one course of everything in terms of NCLEX [National Council Licensure Examination], or why they would like to spend more time in one clinical area with more coursework.

Moving from unit to unit, from population to population, can severely influence some students' entry into practice by making it difficult to feel "a part of" and to understand how to interact with the culture of nursing in terms of one patient population. Through dialogue that must be based on seeking out all voices in the situation and which influences everyone involved, students in their own personal ways make decisions about *what* to take *when* in a *way* meaningful to them. Teachers, with students and clinicians, could decide on the types and limit of choices available, and students could become involved and develop their own curriculum. This is a new, practical approach to be tested. I speak now not of offering students two electives in four years, I suggest requiring only two courses, with all other choices being electives.

The Teacher-as-Learner

Importantly, these activities point to a way for teachers to be learners. Teachers engaging in hermeneutic inquiry in which they continually find themselves addressing difficult questions that have meaning for them in the context of teaching reflect the teacher-as-learner. The nature of education as ontology and not epistemology occurs when the students are so engaged in what is being discussed that no one takes a note! The teacher moves from being an information giver and facilitator to the explorer of meanings with students—their understandings of their experiences. Hermeneutic inquiry necessitates dialogue in which students come to understand what it means to be a nurse-teacher and vice-versa. We need to develop a pedagogy that is *attentive* to the histories, futures, and experiences that nursing students and teachers bring with them to school, as well as the experiences of nurses and our patients.

Instead of lecturing, discussing nursing interventions, and assuming students will do their own review of physiology, pathophysiology, and medical treatment, teachers could present patient paradigms—the lived experiences of people who were cared for by expert nurses. These would not be case studies specifically constructed to point out what the teacher wants to teach (although this can always be included), but rather *lived experiences* in which students come to think about and experience the complexities and incongruencies of nursing practice.

The struggle for the teacher then is to learn how students develop meanings for their practice out of the experiences teachers provide. This problem of trying to understand how and what students are learning will be a problem that will help all teachers be forever learners. Students and nursing knowledge will always change, and so must the teacher. In this manner, the teacher both shapes and is shaped by learning.

Secondly, in this role, teachers are in the world through their continual rebirth of the struggle to understand. Perhaps the primordial being of the teacher—prior to the understanding of teacher as information teller, facilitator of learning, evaluator—is teacher-as-learner. A teacher should be in the world learningly; to be open, always, to new possibilities, constantly transforming and being transformed. In this openness, teaching becomes learning, learning is hearing as in dialogue (not listening), and teaching is the struggle to understand. It is a moving-into-nearness; becoming what we are so close to, always, already; and seeking to and being in a way to understand that which is on the one hand so familiar, and on the other hand an abyss of nearness. In this way, by our studying the lived experiences of teachers and by reflecting on our own teaching practice, we are not studying teaching but rather learning. (Think of those times you've had with students that you'll never forget—because they taught you something about what it means to be a teacher.) Increasing our understanding of the practice of teaching will contribute greatly to the development of a new pedagogy for nursing.

CONCLUSION

Where has this free play led us? I would now like to raise some issues for our discussion as we struggle to understand more about our practice of teaching and the nature of nursing education as teaching and learning.

This revolution should not be one of a few voices "teaching" and "showing new possibilities" to others. Rather, it should consist of multiple voices, coming together, examining the concerns we share in the contexts of our present teaching practices. This will provoke us to think further, for precisely therein lies the pedagogical horizon for us. If our dialogues with each other end in riddles rather than in answers, we have not been misled. As Heidegger has argued, "The task is to see the riddle" (Heidegger, 1971b, p. 79).

How can we empower students and have them join us? How can we include our clinical colleagues in the revolution? How can we become politically active in changing the structures within nursing that act as barriers (such as aspects of the accreditation process), transform education, and explore alternatives? How and where can we each use our influence to exert pressure to attain these changes? We also need to look at the ways in which the structural forces outside the immediacy of our schools of nursing construct the objective conditions within which schools function. We need to have dialogue around educational policies as a part of evaluating schools of nursing.

I call on you to join the Society for Research in Nursing Education, a Council of the National League for Nursing, and to attend the annual scientific meeting. This revolution needs strong links between the practitioners and researchers of nursing education. Practitioners must inform researchers of the dilemmas that confront them, and researchers must translate to practitioners the solutions, new possibilities, and approaches that emerge from research. In this way, those in the practice of education can exchange ideas with those involved with research findings and knowledge. New approaches to nursing education are beginning to emerge (Bevis & Watson, in press). In these activities, we must include student and clinicians. It is timely for us to unite; to care because we are teachers, clinicians, students, and patients concerned about preparing the caretakers of the future.

Central to this dialogue are understandings of politics and power. The dialectical exploration of the political ideologies implicit in our current practices and the historical interpretations of the background in which we currently practice in nursing education by critical theorists and feminist scholars are part of the unveiling process (Allen, 1985; Giroux, 1988b; Weiler, 1988). We need to make visible the nature of teachers' work—the conditions under which teachers labor (Apple, 1986). Each of us engaged in the struggle to create, defend, and extend the discourse of preparing future caretakers has an essential role to play.

We must also move beyond the language of critique and domination and develop a language of possibilities—a language of nursing education. Hermeneutic studies, like the one we are conducting here, will make visible the practice of teaching in nursing.

We have not explored graduate and doctoral education in this chapter, but the implications of the revolution are enormous. Functional coursework in nursing education will change as we begin to uncover the practical knowledge of teaching in nursing. As the evolution of teaching skills in nursing becomes understood, new possibilities for teaching practicums emerge. Students, least encumbered with educational dogma, often retain the new and needed insights.

If the revolution is calling into question behavioral education and concomitantly our present way of thinking about teaching and learning, it is imperative that we keep ourselves open to new possibilities. For all of us to be learners is for us to struggle with dilemmas that confront us. I have proposed hermeneutical phenomenology as a fundamental way—a way station—to help us understand the nature of teaching while we await and create new approaches. But we also need to have dialogue and research about the meaning of structures, both within and outside our schools, that are part of our very being.

Attention to the societal content, the nature of our practice as clinicians and teachers, and concern that is ultimately rooted in nursing practice will unite us. In this way, we live the continual rebirth of our struggle to understand.

REFERENCES

Allen, D. (1985). Nursing research and social control: Alternative models of science that emphasize understanding and emancipation. *Image, 17*(2), 58–64.

Apple, M. (1986). *Teachers and texts: A political economy of class and gender relations in education.* New York: Routledge & Kegan Paul.

Benner, P. (1984). *From novice to expert: Excellence and power in clinical nursing practice.* Menlo Park, CA: Addison-Wesley.

Benner, P., & Tanner, C. (1987, January). Clinical judgment: How expert nurses use intuition. *American Journal of Nursing, 87*(1), 23–31.

Benner, P., & Wrubel, J. (1989). *The primacy of caring: Stress and coping in health and illness.* Menlo Park, CA: Addison-Wesley.

Bevis, E., & Watson, J. (in press). *A new direction for curriculum development for professional nursing: A paradigm shift from training to education.* New York: National League for Nursing.

Diekelmann, N. (1986). *Dialogue and meaning: Essential knowledge for the professional nurse curriculum.* Unpublished manuscript, American Association of Colleges of Nursing Pew Project.

Diekelmann, N. (1988). *From layperson to novice nurse: The lived experiences of nursing students.* Unpublished manuscript, University of Wisconsin, School of Nursing, Madison.

Diekelmann, N., Allen, D., & Tanner, C. (in press). *The National League for Nursing criteria for appraisal of baccalaureate programs: A critical hermeneutical analysis.* New York: National League for Nursing.

Feinburg, W. (1983). *Understand education: Toward a reconstruction of educational inquiry.* New York: Cambridge University Press.

Giroux, H. (1988a). *Teachers as intellectuals: Toward a critical pedagogy of learning.* South Hadley, MA: Bergin & Garvey.

Giroux, H. (1988b). *Schooling and the struggle for public life: Critical pedagogy in the modern age.* Minneapolis: University of Minnesota Press.

Greene, M. (1988). *The dialectic of freedom.* New York: Teachers College Press, Columbia University.

Heidegger, M. (1962). *Being and time* (J. Macquarrie & E. Robinson, Trans.). New York: Harper & Row.

Heidegger, M. (1971a). *On the way to language* (P. Hertz, Trans.). New York: Harper & Row.

Heidegger, M. (1971b). *Poetry, language, thought* (A. Hofstadter, Trans.). New York: Harper & Row.

Kliebard, H. (1977). The Tyler rationale. In W. Pinar (Ed.), *Curriculum and evaluation* (pp. 56–67). Berkeley, CA: McCutchan.

Magee, B. (1987). *The great philosophers: An introduction to western philosophy. Dialogue 12: Husserl, Heidegger and Modern Existentialism with Hubert Dreyfus.* London: BBC Books.

May, W. (1988). Adversarialism in America. In C. H. Reynolds & R. V. Norman (Eds.), *Community in America: The challenge of habits of the heart* (pp. 185–201). Berkeley: University of California Press.

Merleau-Ponty, M. (1962). *The phenomenology of perception* (C. Smith, Trans.). London: Routledge & Kegan Paul.

Polkinghorne, D. (1988). *Narrative knowing and the human sciences.* Albany: State University of New York Press.

Ricouer, P. (1984–1986). *Time and narrative* (Vols. 1, 2) (K. McLaughlin & D. Pellauer, Trans.). Chicago: University of Chicago Press.

Shor, I. (1986). *Culture wars: School and society in the conservative restoration, 1969–1984.* London: Routledge & Kegan Paul.

Tanner, C., Padrick, K. P., Westfall, U. E., & Puzier, D. J. (1987). Diagnostic reasoning strategies of nurses and nursing students. *Nursing Research, 36,* 358–363.

Weber, S. (1986). The nature of interviewing. *Phenomenology & Pedagogy, 4*(2), 65–70.

Weiler, K. (1988). *Women teaching for change: Gender, class and power.* South Hadley, MA: Bergin & Garvey.

4

Faculty–Student Relationships: Catalytic Connection

Gloria M. Clayton, EdD, RN
Joyce P. Murray, MSN, RN

REVOLUTION AS OPPORTUNITY

What is the right thing to do when in the midst of a revolution? The titles of the 1987 and 1988 National Conferences on Nursing Education included the hard-to-ignore phrase, "Curriculum Revolution." How can you and I participate lest we be accused of "wasting time in the revolution" as the currently popular Tracy Chapman ballad describes? We can act on several levels.

The first, and perhaps most important, action is to maintain optimism. As Watson (1985) says:

> For perhaps the first time in its scientific development, nursing has recently had the opportunity to explore its own heritage, become recommitted to nursing values, goals, and philosophies, and explore research methods and options consistent with prevailing views about the nature of nursing. In so doing, nursing scholars and clinicians have begun to admit openly that an inconsistency or anomaly has existed and continues to exist between the medical tradition and/or natural science paradigm and the nature of nursing. (p. 19)

Another level of action is our scholarly contribution. This will be unique to our individual talents and expertise. It may be in the form of theory development, inquiry, or wise consumption of the new literature. All are valid pursuits critical to our successes.

But what can we do in the context of our daily professional lives? There are approximately 20,000 nurses teaching in schools of nursing

(Vaughn & Johnson, 1981), all of whom are struggling with students in both classroom and clinical settings in the midst of a revolution that Capra (1982) calls a "turning point" or a compelling vision of a new reality. At last year's conference, Donley (1987) indicated in her opening address that the mandate for change is nothing less than the need for a new world view on health. The magnitude of initiating this type of change makes it quite tempting for the 20,000 of us in class and clinical to despair and do nothing. The response of a professor of urban values at New York University upon his resignation is common. He stated: "I don't have anything to say anymore. I don't think anybody does. When a problem becomes too difficult, you lose interest" (Capra, 1982, p. 25).

Feeling pulled in many directions, we concluded that the primary opportunity for impact is the relationship formed with each and every student. This chapter reviews the literature found to be helpful in making decisions about these relationships and the interactions which create them. Faculty and student interactions are determined by what is believed by those involved about learning and teaching. Reviews of learning, teaching, and faculty and student interaction are followed by findings from our research.

ATTAINING KNOWLEDGE

The behaviorist's definition of learning includes changes in behavior as a measure of learning, whereas the Gestalt psychologists define learning in terms of reorganization of the learner's perceptual or psychological world (Bigge, 1976). Reviews of recent literature revealed a frequently used phrase—"ways of knowing"—which is closely related to learning. If an individual learns, how do they learn or know? Eisner (1985), editor of *Learning and Teaching the Ways of Knowing,* explores the ideas of form, coherence, knowledge of, knowledge through, and stimulation. He states that "curriculum is a mind-altering device and, when content and tasks are selected, the teacher has defined the kind of mental skills that will be cultivated" (p. 34).

A five-year phenomenological study conducted by Belenky, Clinchy, Goldberger, and Tarule (1986) offers a model of *Women's Ways of Knowing.* This study has major implications for nursing, whose membership is 95–98 percent female. An intensive interview/case study approach was used to explore women's experiences and problems as learners and knowers, as well as to review their past histories for changing concepts of the self and relationships with others. To assure diversity and strengthen the importance of the findings, 135 women with varied demographic characteristics were interviewed. Ninety were enrolled in academic institutions and 45 women were from family agencies that dealt with clients seeking information about, or assistance with, parenting. The first phase of the analyses centered on the segment of the interview which was designed to elicit information on the women's assumptions about the nature of truth, knowledge, and authority. Blind coding and contextual analyses techniques, used to analyze the data, resulted in the grouping of women's perspectives of knowing into five major epistemological categories:

1. Silence—a position in which women view themselves as mindless and voiceless and subject to the whims of external authority
2. Received knowledge—a perspective from which women see themselves as being capable of receiving and reproducing knowledge from the all-knowing external authorities, but not capable of creating knowledge on their own
3. Subjective knowledge—a perspective from which truth and knowledge are conceived as personal, private, and subjectively known or intuited
4. Procedural knowledge—a position in which women are invested in learning and applying objective procedures of obtaining and communicating knowledge
5. Constructed knowledge—a position in which women view all knowledge as contextual, experience themselves as creators of knowledge, and value both subjective and objective strategies for knowing (Belenky et al., 1986, p. 15)

An important finding of this research is the assumption that personal development will occur as a result of the educational process. Clearly our students need to function at a level of subjective knowledge or procedural knowledge when they begin practice. Educators can assist women in developing authentic voices of their own. This can be accomplished by focusing on "connected teaching" that emphasizes connectedness over separation, understanding over assessment, collaboration over debate, and allows time for knowledge to emerge from firsthand experiences, while encouraging students to evolve their own patterns of work based on the presented problems.

Carper (1978) described fundamental patterns of knowing in nursing, which were identified from an analysis of the conceptual and syntactical structure of nursing knowledge. They are distinguished according to logical type of meaning and are designated as (a) empirics, the science of nursing; (b) esthetics, the art of nursing; (c) the component of personal knowledge in nursing; and (d) ethics, the component of moral knowledge in nursing. As Carper states, "the body of knowledge that serves as the rationale for nursing practice has patterns, forms, and structures that serve as horizons of expectations and characteristic ways of thinking about phenomena" (p. 14). Approaching learning experiences from this framework broadens perspectives with which one can consider the phenomena of health and illness.

A major contribution to the literature on learning was the 1979 report of a learning project sponsored by the Club of Rome, written by authors from socialist and third-world countries, as well as the West. The purpose of this project was to focus primarily on the human element in relation to such global problems as energy, communication, cultural identity, and the arms race. Because the human being will be the key to the world's future, the world must come to understand two critical points. Humanity is rapidly moving toward a crossroads where there will be no room for mistakes, and, secondly, the vicious cycle of increasing complexity and lagging understanding must be broken while it is still possible to exert human influence and control over our destiny and future. The human gap, the distance between increasing complexity and the capacity to cope, and bridging the gap through learning are examined in this report. In light of this, Botkin, Elmandjra, and Malitza (1979) define learning as:

> . . . an approach to knowledge and to life that emphasizes human initiative. It encompasses the acquisition and practice of new methodologies, new skills, new attitudes, and new values to live in a changing world. Learning is the process of preparing to deal with new situations. It may occur consciously or often unconsciously, usually from experiencing real-life situations, although simulated or imagined situations can also induce learning. (p. 8)

Every individual in the world, whether or not in an educational setting, is learning; however, probably no one is learning at the level, intensity, and speed needed to cope with the complexities faced in modern life. The authors describe two types of learning, one that is presently occurring in society and one that society must pursue for long-term survival.

Maintenance learning is traditionally found in societies today, and is described as the acquisition of fixed outlooks, methods, and rules for dealing with known and recurring situations (Botkin et al., 1979, p. 10). Problem solving is geared toward given problems, and it is this type of learning that only maintains an existing system or established way of life.

Innovative learning has two primary features—anticipation and participation. It is this type of learning that will prepare individuals to act collectively in situations. Anticipatory learning prepares individuals to use techniques such as forecasting, simulations, scenarios, and models. It encourages consideration of trends, planning, evaluating future consequences and possible side effects of present decisions, and recognizing the far-reaching side effects. Participation involves more than the formal sharing of decisions. It is characterized by an attitude of cooperation, dialogue, and empathy. It means keeping communication open and constantly testing the operating rules and values, while retaining the relevant and rejecting the obsolete. There are questions to be raised in reaction to this report. What are the implications for learning in the institutions of higher learning? What kinds of learning are needed to meet the demands of nursing in the future? What kinds of learning experiences will provide students with the types of learning they need?

TEACHING

Chickering (1969) generates two hypotheses related to types of teaching experiences. Hypothesis A states: "When few electives are offered, when books and print are the sole objects of study, when teaching is by lecture, when evaluation is frequent and competitive, ability to memorize is fostered. Sense of competence, freeing of interpersonal relationships, and development of autonomy, and identity, and purpose are not" (p. 148). Conversely, Hypothesis B states: "When choice and flexibility are offered, when direct experiences are called for, when teaching is by discussion, and when evaluation involves frequent communication concerning the substance of behavior and performance, the ability to analyze and synthesize is fostered, as are sense of competence, freeing of interpersonal relationships, and development of autonomy, identity, and purpose" (p. 148). Chickering provides data to support his belief that curriculum, teaching, and evaluation are linked together and that the approach to each has implications for the development of the student in the areas of intellectual competence, cognitive behaviors, sense of competence, development of emotional and instrumental independence, identity, interpersonal relationships, and clarifying purposes.

The research of Benner (1984) is greatly impacting teaching as well. The purpose of the study was to discover knowledge embedded in clinical practice, and to determine the differences in clinical performances and situational appraisals of neophyte and expert nurses. To obtain data, paired interviews were conducted with beginning nurses and nurses recognized for their expertise. The pairs were interviewed separately about patient situations they had shared which were relevant to them. The aim was to determine if distinguishable differences existed between novice and expert descriptions of the same clinical incident. Additionally, 51 experienced nurse clinicians, 11 new nurse graduates, and 5 senior nursing students were interviewed and observed to further delineate and describe characteristics of nurse performance at different stages of skill acquisition (Benner, 1984, p. 14–15). Utilizing the Dreyfus model of skill acquisition combined with interviews and observations, the performance characteristics at each level of development were described and identified in general terms as the teaching–learning needs at each of the five levels (novice, advanced beginner, competent, proficient, and expert).

Several implications for types of learning experiences and education of professional nurses came out of this study.

1. A situation-based interpretive approach to nursing care is more effective than the linear nursing process model currently being utilized. This linear process model can actually obscure knowledge embedded in clinical nursing practice.
2. Strategies which include content, context, and function are necessary to incorporate the relational aspects of nursing.
3. The accomplishments and characteristics of expert nurse performance can be observed and described in narrative, interpretive form.
4. Exemplar cases of nursing practice offer the advantages of identifying nursing competencies that include actual performance demands, resources, and constraints and provide a rich description of nursing practice.
5. Educational nursing programs must provide the background knowledge necessary for advanced skill acquisition. Descriptions of actual nursing practice can provide a basis for realistic curriculum planning.
6. Understanding the process of acquiring advanced knowledge and skills will teach students and graduates how to go about becoming an expert practitioner (Benner, 1984).

Amidon and Flanders (1967) describe a system for analyzing the classroom verbal behavior of teachers and students. This system delineates three categories: teacher talk, student talk, and silence or confusion. Teacher talk has two subdivisions: indirect and direct. Indirect teacher talk behaviors are categorized into four observational categories: (a) accepting of feeling, (b) praising or encouraging, (c) accepting of ideas, and (d) asking questions. Direct teacher behaviors include: (a) lecturing, (b) giving directions, and (c) criticizing or justifying authority. (Relating this to Chickering's work, indirect teacher talk would be related to Hypothesis B.) The two categories for student behaviors are: (a) responding to teacher, and (b) initiating talk. Silence or confusion would naturally lead to the least desirable (and most frustrating) situation, and should be avoided at all cost.

Several nursing studies provide guidance for teaching strategies and student–instructor relationships. Griffith and Bakanauskas (1983) compared the student–instructor relationship to the therapeutic relationship of nurse–client. They indicated that students benefit from a relationship that provides open, honest communication based on trust and support. They also found that when nurses are involved in such a relationship, they more readily learn the essential therapeutic approaches. Professional socialization, self-actualization, self-fulfillment, and self-concept are also effected by interpersonal relationships along with the abilities of the nursing instructor to meet the students' learning needs. Caring attitudes demonstrated by a respected instructor who acknowledges students' strengths and weaknesses are significant to students' lives and learning. Griffith and Bakanauskas also provided teaching strategies that could facilitate interpersonal growth and learning in this study. Wang and Blumberg (1983) researched interaction techniques of nursing faculty in the clinical area. Observations were grouped into either high- or low-level qualities. Low level interactions included asking leading or direct questions, summarizing statements, and verbal exchange of facts and procedures. High level interactions of faculty allowed students to analyze, synthesize, evaluate, compare, and contrast.

Three recent nursing studies support the importance of faculty practice to quality of teaching. Kramer, Plifron, and Organek (1986) studied 134 baccalaureate students and 14 faculty. Their work confirmed that students who worked with faculty who were also engaged in practice scored higher in autonomy, self-concept, self-esteem, locus of control, and professional role behavior than did students that lacked access to such faculty. This study was based on Bandura's social learning theory and the premise that persons learn under the following conditions:

1. The learner either directly or vicariously observes a model and the consequences of the model's behavior.
2. The learner has the opportunity to practice the behaviors he or she observed.
3. The learner imitates models who are perceived to be expert, competent, or socially powerful.
4. Reinforcement is paramount in the acquisition process and most instrumental when the model, rather than the modeler, perceives reward.

Another study using Bandura's work supports the importance of clinical competence. Cooper (1982) queried 75 students on the importance of faculty role model behaviors. The behaviors were categorized as nursing behaviors, teaching behaviors, or personal behaviors. The nursing behaviors were deemed most critical by students for their learning.

The final study determined the effect of a preceptorship experience on role socialization (Clayton, Broome, & Ellis, in press). Two groups, one having a preceptorship experience in the final quarter of their baccalaureate program (n = 33), and one having the traditional course (n = 33), participated in the study. Both groups completed Schwerian's Six-Dimension Scale of Nursing Performance on three testing occasions; prior to the course, immediately following the course, and six months after graduation. There was a significant relationship between group and time; the preceptor group at the six month follow-up scored significantly higher on four of the six subscales as well as on the overall socialization instrument. The study of intuition, although very new, stresses the importance of intuition in decision making in clinical practice. In Benner's 1984 study, subjects repeatedly referred to a "gut feeling" as influencing their decisions. Rew (1988) explored intuitive experiences with 56 nurses. The findings emphasized the importance of intuition and revealed themes consistent with other literature on intuition. Nurse educators are beginning to recognize the importance of teaching and valuing intuitive skill. Reinforcement of this skill needs to be delineated.

Advisement, an often neglected teaching responsibility, was recently highlighted in a White paper on Undergraduate Education developed at the University of Pennsylvania (Student Committee on Undergraduate Education, 1985). The paper describes critical components of a successful advising system.

> The advising system must allow each student adequate time for self-definition. By verbally clarifying needs and interests in the advising situation, providing sufficient access to all available resources, and guiding the student to course choices that further aid such clarification, advising can better equip students to find and take full advantage of the academic path that best fits these interests. Because the development of attitudes and interests which influence decision making are reflected in changes in students' chosen curricular, academic, and career goals, advising must be prepared to deal with all stages of redefinition and choice the student might encounter in four years. Individual advising is successful when students understand why they make the choices they do, are encouraged to clarify needs and interests upon which they can base their decision, and feel free to redefine their goals if necessary. Students do not go to an advisor to hear them read the catalog; it takes responsive encouragement to guide students as they turn their ideas into realities. (p. 21)

A final area contributing to the body of literature on teaching is working on caring. Two schools which have incorporated this into their curricula are the University of Colorado School of Nursing, which has designed a curriculum based on humanism and caring, and Georgia Southern College, which uses caring as the conceptual framework for their undergraduate curriculum.

Clayton and Murray's (1987) study describes caring experiences among faculty and student dyads. They investigated the phenomena of caring between baccalaureate nursing students and faculty. A goal of nursing is to help persons gain a higher degree of harmony within the mind, body, and soul which generates self-knowledge, self-reverence, self-healing, and self-care processes while allowing increasing diversity (Watson, 1985). This goal is, in part, achieved through the unique relationship that the nurse enters with a client. In a clinical discipline, this relationship is most effectively taught through modeling the preferred nurse–client behaviors via the faculty–student relationship.

Watson's (1985) philosophy and theory of caring guide the selection of methodology and analyses for this research. Using a phenomenological interview, 20 nursing students from 2 programs were interviewed regarding their interaction with a faculty member. The students identified a transpersonal caring occasion and described it in terms of thoughts, feelings, behaviors, and meaning. The involved faculty member was interviewed to ascertain her perspective of the occasion. Additionally, the student–faculty dyad was observed 3 times in a clinical setting. Using grounded theory, the interviews and field notes were analyzed. Recurring themes from the pilot data (n = 10 students and 4 faculty) supported Watson's (1985) theory of caring transactions. A portion of the data set also provided a list of faculty behaviors perceived by students as either caring or noncaring. This discrimination is useful for developing teaching strategies and learning activities.

In a gerontology elective course developed by Clayton (1987) and designed according to Watson's (1985) carative factors, the primary objective was upon increasing awarenesses and developing positive attitudes. Students are introduced to the theories of carative factors with the focus of the remaining classwork upon self-analyses and group discussions. An extensive and diverse "menu" of didactic and experimental learning activities involving older adults is provided, from which each student selects options. To ensure maximum opportunity for pursuit of individual interest, the student may also design other learning options with faculty guidance and approval. Class time focuses on exchanges related to field experiences, examination of stereotypic myths of aging, and discussion of feelings and insights about aging that arise within the group. Options for field experiences include planned activities within community agencies, such as Alzheimer's Support Groups, meal and other aggregation facilities, and viewing contemporary films that feature age-related scenarios. Each student en ers personal insights gained from day-to-day glimpses of life that have implications for the elderly into a daily log. Pre- and posttesting, using Palmore's Facts About Aging Tool and Kogan's Attitude Toward Old People Scale, has demonstrated that the students' attitudes and knowledge about aging improved significantly during the participation in the course.

Clearly, changes in philosophy, curriculum design, and instruction lie ahead. These changes will necessitate reconceptualization of faculty–student relationships and a broader repertoire of interactions. While at this point it is impossible to predict precisely what the future holds, we trust in the genius of many of our colleagues, plus our collective wisdom, to create an optimistic future for nursing. This mandate for change is our opportunity to ensure nursing's best possible future.

REFERENCES

Amidon, E. J., & Flanders, W. (1967). Interaction analysis as a feedback system. In E. J. Amidon & J. B. Haugh (Eds.), *Interaction analysis: Theory, research and application* (pp. 121–140). Reading, MA: Addison-Wesley.

Belenky, M. F., Clinchy, B. Mc., Goldberger, N., & Tarule, J. (1986). *Women's ways of knowing.* New York: Basic.

Benner, P. (1984). *From novice to expert.* Menlo Park, CA: Addison-Wesley.

Bigge, M. L. (1976). *Learning theories for teachers* (3rd ed.). New York: Harper & Row.

Botkin, T. W., Elmandjra, M. & Malitza, M. (1979). *No limits to learning.* Elmsford, NY: Pergamon.

Capra, F. (1982). *The turning point.* New York: Bantam.

Carper, B. A. (1978). Fundamental patterns of knowing in nursing. *Advances in Nursing Science, 1*(1), 13–23.

Chickering, A. W. (1969). *Education and identity.* San Francisco: Jossey-Bass.

Clayton, G. M., Broome, M., & Ellis, L. (in press). Relationship between a preceptorship experience and role socialization of graduate nurses. *Journal of Nursing Education.*

Clayton, G., & Murray, J. (1987). *Caring in faculty/student dyad.* Presented at the International Conference on Nursing Education, Cardiff, Wales.

Cooper, G. (1982). *Characteristics students view as important in nurse faculty role models.* Unpublished master's thesis, University of Mississippi, Oxford, MS. (EDRA Document No. 246793.)

Donley, Sr. R. (1987). Opening address, *Fourth National Conference on Nursing Education,* Philadelphia, PA.

Eisner, E. W. (1985). *The educational imagination* (2nd ed.). New York: Macmillan.

Griffith, T. W., & Bakanauskas, A. J. (1983). Student-instructor relationships in nursing education. *Journal of Nursing Education, 22*(3), 104–107.

Kramer, M., Plifron, C., & Organek, N. (1986). Effects of faculty practice on students learning outcomes. *Journal of Professional Nursing, 2*(5), 289–301.

Rew, L. (1988). Intuition in decision-making. *Image: Journal of Nursing Scholarship, 20*(3), 150–154.

Student Committee on Undergraduate Education white paper on undergraduate education. (1985). University of Pennsylvania, PA. (EDRS Document No. ED 260 622.)

Vaughn, J. C., & Johnson, W. L. (1981). *Nursing data book, 1981.* New York: National League for Nursing.

Wang, A. M., & Blumberg, P. (1983). A study on interaction techniques of nursing faculty in the clinical area. *Journal of Nursing Education, 22*(3), 144–151.

Watson, J. (1985). *Nursing: Human science and human care.* Norwalk, CT: Appleton-Century-Crofts.

5

Clinical Teaching: Paradoxes and Paradigms

Carol A. Lindeman, PhD, RN, FAAN

The topic of clinical teaching often produces feelings of dilemma. We know it is a very significant educational component of entry level programs, yet we know very little about effective use of the clinical laboratory. At the same time that the clinical competence of the nurse is taking on new meanings and greater importance, the clinical laboratory settings seen as essential for developing clinical competence are changing in ways that detract from their suitability for use by entry level programs. The Delphi study of priorities and assumptions in research in nursing education is evident in the extent of nurse educators' concerns about clinical teaching (Tanner & Lindeman, 1987). Six of the top ten research priorities related to clinical teaching identified in this study are:

1. What method of instruction best develops clinical problem solving skills at baccalaureate and master's levels?
2. What is the most effective approach to teaching clinical nursing skills?
3. What clinical teaching strategies are more conducive to the development of professional qualities; e.g., critical thinking, accountability, change agent?
4. What types of clinical performance evaluation strategies are most reliable and valid?
5. What factors enhance the transfer of didactic learning into clinical practice?

6. What factors in clinical experience (e.g., number of hours, rotations, faculty–student ratios) are associated with the level of performance at graduation?

This chapter examines the question of clinical teaching from three perspectives—historical, contemporary, and future. In section one, the 1937 *Curriculum guide for schools of nursing* is used to create a context for identifying the paradoxes in clinical teaching. In section two, current literature and personal experience are used to place each paradox in a contemporary framework. Section three includes recommendations for future paradigms.

HISTORICAL PERSPECTIVE

A Curriculum Guide for Schools of Nursing (1937) states that the function of nursing schools is to select students who show particular aptitude for nursing; to provide suitable opportunities for them to learn to adjust to the professional situations they are likely to meet; and to guide their learning in such a way that they will be able to give efficient service to society as professional nurses, enjoy the satisfactions that come from such service, and attain the fullest growth of which they are capable. Clearly the schools' main function at this point was to prepare students for the real world of nursing practice, with "practice" defined as the providing of direct care.

The Committee on Curriculum (authors of *A Curriculum Guide for Schools of Nursing*) believed the curriculum should reflect the activities, functions, duties, and responsibilities of those working in the field. They refer to a compilation of several different lists of detailed activities totaling about 800 items. The goal of nursing education was to produce a professional nurse competent to provide the following tasks and services to patients requiring care in the hospital and community:

- Observing and recognizing symptoms, conditions, and causes—mental, physical, and social (73 activities)
- Carrying on curative nursing procedures (221 activities)
- Carrying on preventive nursing procedures (42 activities)
- Creating and maintaining proper psychological atmosphere (48 activities)
- Preparing and administering diets (33 activities)
- Giving medications and preparing solutions (49 activities)
- Assisting physician in examining patients, giving treatments, and making diagnostic tests (48 activities)

- Checking, recording, receiving and giving reports, and caring for records (41 activities)
- Creating and maintaining proper physical environment and supervising other workers to this end (38 activities)
- Teaching measures to conserve health and to restore health (143 activities)
- Cooperating with family, hospital personnel, and health and social agencies in the interests of patient and of community (45 activities)
- Giving attention to the patient's possessions and protecting his interests (17 activities)

The Committee summarized this, stating that:

> Therefore, so far as the education of professional nurses is concerned, they must in any case know all the activities thoroughly and in addition, be able to analyze nursing situations, know what type of nursing activities are required, plan and carry out a well-coordinated program of nursing care (with or without assistants), and evaluate the results.

The Committee reasoned that because nursing students are giving professional service (under supervision) during most of their period of preparation, their skill level must be higher than that of students in other professional schools. They recommended that nursing students receive 1100–1200 hours of systematic instruction and 4400–5000 hours of nursing practice during their program. Converting this into aggregate credit hours, the recommended balance was approximately 43 percent instruction and 57 percent practice. The Committee recommended that theory and practical experience should run parallel and should be integrated, not merely correlated. Teaching strategies are briefly described with the notation that they are applicable in both the classroom and clinical setting. The supervisory role of the instructor in the clinical setting is mentioned frequently.

Reflections on this review of the origins of current nursing education combined with nursing street knowledge yields several generalizations germane to clinical teaching:

1. Experience in the clinical setting is a very significant component of entry-level nursing education.
2. The student should experience realities of nursing in the clinical setting.
3. The instructor is also the student's supervisor.
4. Students learn by providing care to patients and families using a problem-solving framework; that care must match the standards set

by the profession. The classroom setting provides the knowledge base that is applied in the clinical setting.

Inherent in these generalizations are the paradoxes of clinical teaching in today's world of nursing education.

CONTEMPORARY FOCUS

Paradox Number One: *The clinical laboratory is an essential component of nursing education, yet it is becoming increasingly difficult to find clinical placements appropriate for entry-level programs.*

There are so many influences on today's nurses that simply could not be foreseen in 1937. Because they are now part of our lives, these factors and their implications cannot be ignored. For example, in 1987 the Division of Nursing (Bureau of Health Professions, Health Resources and Services Administration, U.S. Department of Health and Human Services) undertook a major project with four regional professional nursing organizations to obtain data which would assess the impact of the prospective payment system on nursing practice and the subsequent implications for undergraduate nursing education. From the reports of that project and the current health care literature, it is clear that the prospective payment system has influenced nursing practice with numerous implications for nursing education. Changes in the acute-care setting include:

1. Decreased lengths of stay, i.e., patients are admitted for a shorter length of time, are sicker during their stay, and are sicker when they are discharged
2. Increased intensity of care, i.e., more patients are treated in other settings so the staff nurse now cares for *only* acutely ill patients (no convalescing or preprocedure patients to balance the workload)
3. Early discharge resulting in increased referrals and teaching activities
4. Increased scope of nursing responsibilities including picking up tasks previously done by licensed practical nurses or ancillary staff such as respiratory therapists
5. Rationing of services based on cost-effectiveness judgments including consideration of legal and ethical issues
6. Increased importance of quality assurance including clinical outcomes
7. A fluctuating census with higher peaks and lower valleys
8. Increased requirements for reimbursement relevant data

Changes in the home health care setting include:

1. An increase in the number of patients referred to home health care; requiring hiring new personnel, extensive staff development, and new program development
2. Use of high technology in the home (ventilator, intravenous and blood transfusions, enteral therapy) requiring 24-hour-a-day, 7-day-a-week service
4. Inconsistent, restrictive, and retroactive reimbursement policies at the federal level
5. Mandatory uniform data collection that requires incredible detail and an inordinant amount of time
5. Mandatory uniform data collection that requires incredible detail and an inordinant amount of time
6. Increased competition among providers
7. An increasing gap between patients' needs and the care reimbursed by Medicare

Changes in the long-term care setting include:

1. Increasing acuity of patients admitted to long-term care
2. Increasing nursing care requirements for patients admitted to long-term care
3. A need for more registered nurses
4. A nursing staff prepared in ethics, health care financing, and the latest technology

The introduction of prospective financing of health care has resulted in countless changes in the nature of nursing practice. Nurses in most, if not all, clinical settings practice under conditions of rationing. There are simply not enough financial and human resources available to provide the necessary care for all of the patients. The nurse must ration the care provided. There was a time when good nursing care was defined as doing everything one knew how to do for every patient you cared for. I call that the nursing imperative definition of good nursing care. Today, good nursing care is defined as providing those services that are cost effective with the concept of "effective" including assessment of outcomes and ethical issues.

In this fast-paced, rapidly changing world of health care delivery, the use of the clinical setting as the clinical laboratory in the education of all health professionals becomes increasingly more difficult. The growing acuity level of most patients now makes the hospital a massive intensive care unit. Changes in demographics have also influenced this setting by filling beds with the frail elderly. Entry-level nursing students are not prepared for the complex medical and nursing requirements of these patients and can hardly be expected to function at the level of the expert nurse clinician. Although the nursing home may now provide clinical experiences more suitable to the entry-level student, its staffing and reimbursement problems may preclude it from serving as a clinical laboratory for many students. Likewise, the reimbursement issues for home health care have forced practice toward only doing what is reimbursable, using less well-prepared nursing personnel, and insisting on very rigid charting practices. This has decreased the value of the home care setting as a clinical laboratory. I believe that as a result of the changes in financing health care, it will become increasingly difficult to find clinical settings with patient populations suitable for entry-level students. This view is supported by nurses in clinical settings.

It seems obvious that the real world of nursing takes greater maturity and knowledge than it did even ten years ago. To place entry-level students in today's clinical setting and expect them to provide care according to long-established standards of the profession is not reasonable. More than ever I believe that we must create clinical laboratories within clinical settings where students are allowed to be students and to learn—not just demonstrate—their practice.

Paradox Number Two: *The clinical laboratory is considered essential because students should learn to function in the real world, yet the current health care delivery system is under attack by the public, legislators, and many health professionals.*

In the 1937 *Curriculum Guide,* nurse educators were cautioned to select clinical settings for student education that were known to have high standards. It was clear that faculty placed students in clinical settings where nursing practice and patient care exemplified what students were to learn. This principle holds true today as well. It is more effective for students to learn where there are positive examples of the behaviors they are learning. How do many of today's clinical settings match that criteria?

A recent editorial in *Nursing Management* (Curtin, 1988) described a nurse who allowed an infant to suffer brain damage. Because the nurse was frustrated with the environment in which she had to practice, she decided to let the patient and doctor suffer the consequences of the doctor's decisions. According to the editor of *Nursing Management,* situations such as these are not rare. The Food and Drug Administration has raised questions about the high incidence of errors made by registered nurses in the use of medical technology. In addition, the Secretary's Commission on Nursing has called attention to the chronic problems of the profession, including low salaries, poor working conditions, having limited authority, being overworked, and lacking in professional stature. Just because a clinical setting is the real world, it may not be the best place to educate students. It may not be the right setting to use to determine competency.

I believe that we create problems for our profession by continuing to use the yardstick of the so-called real world of nursing practice for learning experiences and evaluating students. Once schooled in those values, practicing nurses are not likely to change.

Paradox Number Three: *The clinical laboratory is a part of the educational program, yet student access to it requires evidence of ability to perform according to professional standards.*

There are two aspects to this paradox. The first aspect relates to the role of the instructor, the second relates to the definition of practice. The paradigm we tend to use in clinical instruction is having one faculty member and an assigned group of 8 to 10 students use a given clinical setting for a set number of days and weeks. The faculty member will have negotiated access to that setting by demonstrating competency, assuring the nursing staff that he or she is accountable for the actions of the students, and that they will provide safe care. In this paradigm, one faculty member is accountable for the care being provided to some 16–20 acutely ill patients; patients that the instructor may barely know and who certainly are not part of his or her own caseload. The instructor is also accountable for the well-being of the students and carries a heavier patient careload than the regular staff. Evaluation rather than learning is given priority.

Virden, Loper-Powers, and Spitzer (undated) surveyed 141 baccalaureate nursing students regarding clinical instructor behaviors that enhanced and hindered the students' self-confidence as nurses. The following six behaviors were identified as very helpful:

- Gives positive feedback
- Encourages the students to ask questions
- Is accepting of students' questions
- Creates a climate in which less than perfect behavior at new skills is acceptable
- Provides opportunities for students' independent action
- Encourages discussion of patient care

Three behaviors were rated as "hinders some" or "hinders very much":

- Gives mostly negative feedback
- Observes the student providing care without warning

- Is present for evaluation (and not instruction or assistance) while observing students providing care

In clinical situations where the instructor is under great stress and must supervise to ensure safe care, it is likely that hindering behaviors will predominate. It is also common for the instructor's stress to be passed along to the students.

The other aspect of this paradox relates to the definition of practice. The word practice has two distinct meanings. One meaning is doing what you know how to do and the second is to learn through experience. The first meaning emphasizes the application of existing knowledge; the second, the knowledge that generates from the situation, from the experience itself. If the student must perform according to existing standards and, therefore, practice is seen as the demonstration of one's ability to apply existing knowledge, little learning relevant to the second meaning of practice will occur. Learning of this latter type is likely to be more important for the rapidly changing world of health care.

Paradox Number Four: *The problem-solving approach used in the clinical laboratory emphasizes the application of scientifically derived knowledge to the individual situation, and thereby minimizes the knowledge generated by the situation. The latter knowledge may be the more important for the clinician.*

If I were to ask you whether you agree or disagree with the following definition of practice, I would predict that the majority of you would agree. Practice is defined as a deliberately planned sequence of actions carried out by highly skilled individuals in response to particularized needs of clients. Schon (1987) calls this view of professional practice "instrumental problem solving," and "technical rationality."

Schon states:

> The professional schools of the modern research university are premised on technical rationality. Their normative curriculum, first adopted in the early decades of the twentieth century as the professions sought to gain prestige by establishing their schools in universities, still embodies the idea that practical competence becomes professional when its instrumental problem solving is grounded in systematic, preferably scientific knowledge. So the normative professional curriculum presents first the relevant basic science, then the relevant applied science, and finally, a practicum in which students are presumed to learn to apply research-based knowledge to the problems of everyday practice.

Schon goes on to say that in the throes of external attack and internal self-doubt, professional educators are questioning two fundamental assumptions: that academic research yields useful professional knowledge, and that the professional knowledge taught in the schools prepares the students for the real world of practice. Awareness of these two gaps undermines confidence in professional education as it is currently conceived. Thoughtful educators have responded in four different ways. Some have defined the problem as one of keeping up with the rapidly changing and proliferating knowledge. Others have focused on aspects of the curriculum, such as ethics, which are currently not addressed adequately. Others see the problem as a need to increase the rigor of the current model and return to former levels of excellence. Still others believe the prevailing conception of professional practice and its relationship to science is flawed and a new epistemology of practice must be created. Schon promotes the fourth response by proposing new conceptions of practice competence and professional knowledge that start from the following premises:

- Inherent in the practice of the professionals we recognize as usually competent is a core of artistry.
- Artistry is an exercise of intelligence, a kind of knowing, though different in crucial respects from our standard model of professional knowledge. It is not inherently mysterious; it is rigorous in its own terms; and we can learn a great deal about it—within what limits, we should treat as an open question—by carefully studying the performance of unusually competent performers.
- In the terrain of professional practice, applied science and research-based technique occupy a critically important though limited territory, bounded on several sides by artistry. There exists an art of problem framing, an art of implementation, and an art of improvisation—all necessary to mediate the use in practice of applied science technique.

Schon calls for changes in professional education to create a "reflective practicum"—a practicum aimed at helping students acquire the kinds of artistry essential to competence in the indeterminate zones of practice.

In a complementary line, Jacobs-Kramer and Chinn (1988) present a model that constructs a perspective on the generation, transmission, and evaluation of knowledge forms other than traditional empirics. They discuss four knowledge patterns: empirical, ethical, personal, and esthetic. They conclude:

> Processes within the creative dimension of esthetics enfold the separate knowledge forms that are exhibited as an ongoing art-act. The art-act of nursing, and not separate knowledge forms, provides an avenue for examination of the credibility of nursing practice. Valid empirics, just ethics, and congruent selves are important, and critical questions within each

knowledge pattern need to be asked and answered. An examination of the art-act that integrates all knowledge patterns as expressed in practice provides a comprehensive, context-sensitive means for enfolding multiple knowledge patterns. This shift toward integration of all knowledge patterns will move nursing away from a quest for structural truth and toward a search for dynamic meaning (Munhall, 1986).

A focus on the art-act toward the evolution of dynamic consensual meaning is to be valued, because it promotes choice and freedom from the constraints of considering only one knowledge pattern as credible. Choice and freedom are values consistent with promotion of health. As nurses exercise the freedom to examine practice as art and analyze all patterns of knowing expressed through practice, their effectiveness as promoters of health will be enhanced.

Tanner (1988), in her address to this conference last year, stated:

> As a beginning nurse educator in the early 1970s, I adopted the prevailing approach to teaching clinical judgment as the nursing process. It provided a clear step-by-step linear approach to nursing judgments, a rational model which encouraged the students to clearly identify their assessment data, their plans stated as patient-centered objectives, their nursing orders and the accompanying scientific rationale, and their evaluation of the effectiveness and efficiency of the plan. I gradually became aware of the fact that while some students could write elegant care plans, these same students lacked flexibility to respond to rapidly changing practice situations, or the practical know-how to truly do the interventions. What I was most keenly aware of was that these students had no sense of salience regarding assessment data. They would collect it, and this practice seemed to get no better with time. Moreover, they seemed to have no ability to extract any meaning from the data.

After reviewing the research literature regarding clinical judgment, Tanner concludes:

> We have much to learn from practice and from experts in practice. Now when I think of curriculum revolution, I do not think of developing more elegant and detailed formal models to be passed on to the next generation of nurses, for them to take and apply to their practice. Rather, I am struggling with ways in which the concerns of practice can truly be addressed by our educational activities, where classroom learning might be the application of practice rather than the other way around.

The conception of nursing practice as the use of the problem-solving nursing process made rigorous by incorporating scientifically derived knowledge reflects an inadequate understanding of practice, the knowledge required in practice, and the dynamic relationship between knowing and doing. Yet this conception of practice is the basis for the organization and evaluation of many, if not most, entry-level programs.

PARADIGMS FOR THE FUTURE

At the Oregon Health Sciences University School of Nursing, we have been actively engaged in developing new innovative paradigms for clinical teaching for the last ten years. I wish we had answers. Instead, we have more questions and more appreciation of the complexities of clinical teaching.

Recommendation One: *Reconceptualize nursing practice giving greater value to the art of nursing, to the unity of knowing and doing, and to a knowledge base that includes the empirical, ethical, personal, and esthetic.*

In 1937, the National League for Nursing Committee on Curriculum was clear that schools of nursing were to prepare students for the real world of nursing practice; practice was conceptualized as the ability to *do* some 800 patient care activities. The current paradigm for clinical instruction reflects a conception of practice that emphasizes research and science as the foundations for practice and the nurse as an instrumental problem solver. Over the years we have attempted to increase the rigor of the problem-solving process through the use of the nursing process, the nursing care plan, nursing diagnosis, and most recently, nursing theory. The current paradigm also reflects a hierarchical view of professional roles, with the researcher superior to the practitioner.

It is clear that the view of nursing practice reflected in the current paradigm for clinical teaching is inconsistent with the realities of today's clinical world. Today's world of nursing practice is characterized by ambiguity, uncertainty, complexity, and rapid change. The practitioner and the patient are not passive beneficiaries of science; they are active in the naming and framing of the problem and in selecting appropriate interventions and responses. It is clear to practitioners that patients and clinical situations do not match the nice, neat boxes associated with the empirical approach.

Nursing is more than doing. In the terms of my friends Bill Dickoff and Pat James, it is "Thought Full" doing (personal communication, January 1984). Thinking and doing interact in a dynamic manner in nursing practice. Nurses are more than technology workers; more than technicians applying science to individuals. Clinical learning should incorporate elements of discovery and innovation. It should build knowledge not just use knowledge.

Paradigms for clinical teaching must reflect:

1. The importance of the art of nursing
2. The importance of the knowledge embedded in the clinical encounter
3. The use of self as a major component of the care process
4. The dynamic relationship of knowing and doing
5. The use of a postexperience reflective practicum rather than the preexperience grill and drill

Recommendation Two: *Reconceptualize the teaching–learning process for clinical instruction as a participatory process model that includes the faculty, clinician, student, and patient.*

The 1937 *Curriculum Guide* emphasized the importance of the supervisory role of the faculty in the clinical setting. In the intervening years, the role of the clinical faculty has been one of both instructor and supervisor. In some situations, the faculty member has been the only instructor/supervisor for the students in his or her clinical group. The faculty member has been fully accountable and responsible for the students' learning and the care delivered. In other situations, the faculty member has shared some of the responsibility but not the accountability with members of the nursing staff.

The current paradigm for clinical instruction is unrealistic in today's clinical world. The expert clinician who knows the patient and is familiar with current technology is an essential participant in the teaching–learning process. However, the involvement of the clinician should be as a full participant in the process. The clinician, faculty, and student should share the accountability and responsibility for the quality of student encounters and patient care. As appropriate, the patient should also be involved in the process.

Recommendation Three: *Be more creative and flexible in the selection and use of the real world clinical setting.*

From reading the 1937 *Curriculum Guide,* I can infer that the clinical setting was the primary if not the only setting for acquiring skill in the practice of nursing at that time. In the intervening years, schools of nursing have developed a variety of laboratories to complement the role of the clinical setting. Faculty identified a number of skills and behaviors that students could learn in a nursing arts laboratory, a learning resources center, and a clinical simulation laboratory. My assumption is that these laboratories developed as a response to increasing complexities in the clinical setting and the desire to create a more favorable learning environment.

The changes in the clinical setting associated with the introduction of the prospective payment system have greatly reduced the role of clinical settings in undergraduate teaching. Paradigms for clinical instruction will have to include use of emerging technology for clinical simulation. Preparing for today's world of nursing practice requires opportunity to develop clinical judgment and problem-solving skills in safe environments where innovation is possible. Students need to have the opportunity to follow patients across settings not previously included (clinic, hospital, nursing home). The timing of when the student is exposed to the "real world," as thought of in 1937 where the student practiced at the level of existing standards, needs to be reconsidered and probably delayed.

Recommendation Four: *Demand that the federal government fund research in nursing education and projects demonstrating innovation in clinical teaching.*

Nurse educators have been very polite as they have tried to secure funds to improve instruction. No one in a position of power seems to feel it is a priority; that is in relation to all the other priorities. I know this from personal experience. Several years ago a colleague and I developed a proposal to explore alternate approaches to clinical teaching including a sound evaluation of the costs. We almost secured the funding but the priorities of the foundation changed. We submitted it to another agency who disagreed with our premise that clinical instruction needed to be improved. A third submission produced the response that the proposal was good but we were doing too much evaluation and should submit elsewhere. The fourth submission resulted in the statement that the evaluation wasn't stringent enough. We gave up!! The proposal is still relevant. The questions have never been addressed.

Congress responds to its constituency. Nurse educators, nursing students, and employers of nurses constitute a large constituency. Think of what could happen if we started a campaign to obtain research dollars for nursing education. Why not ride on the coat tails of the nursing shortage and declining enrollments and have nursing education research dollars become a part of Title VIII of the Public Health Service Act?

We know the need for research and demonstration projects. Let's take the next step in the democratic process. Let's articulate that need and propose how Congress can help.

PARADIGMS FOR THE FUTURE

Clinical teaching is clearly one paradox after another. Students in our undergraduate program believe it is the most important part of their program; they are also more dissatisfied with that part of the program than any other. Faculty try to improve the effectiveness of clinical teaching but there are no easy solutions and some potential solutions exceed their authority. We know the issues require more than changing our rhetoric or the trappings surrounding clinical teaching. The issues are the fundamentals. What is nursing? What is knowledge? How do you change lay people into professional practitioners? Let us approach this challenge with the vision of a rainbow. Let's legitimize all of the colors in it and let's use every one.

REFERENCES

Committee on Curriculum of the National League of Nursing Education. (1937). *A curriculum guide for schools of nursing.* New York: Author.

Curtin, L. L. (1988, November). Editorial opinion. *Nursing Management, 19*(11), 7.

Jacobs-Kramer, M. K., & Chinn, P. L. (1988). Perspectives on knowing: A model of nursing knowledge. *Scholarly Inquiry for Nursing Practice: An International Journal,* 2(2), 129–140.

Munhall, P. A. (1986). Methodological issues in nursing research: Beyond a wax apple. *Advances in Nursing Science, 8*(3), 1–5.

Schon, D. A. (1987). *Educating the reflective practitioner: Toward a new design for teaching and learning in the professions.* San Francisco: Jossey-Bass.

Tanner, C. A., & Lindeman, C. A. (1987). Research in nursing education: Assumptions and priorities. *Journal of Nursing Education, 26,* 50–60.

Tanner, C. A. (1988). Curriculum revolution: The practice mandate. In *Curriculum Revolution: Mandate for Change* (pp. 201–216). New York: National League for Nursing.

U.S. Department of Health and Human Services, Public Health Service, Health Resources and Services Administration. (1988). *Impact of DRG's on Nursing: Report of the Western Institute of Nursing.* Springfield, VA: Author.

U.S. Department of Health and Human Services. (1988). *Secretary's Commission on Nursing: Interim Report Executive Summary.* Author.

Virden, S. F., Loper-Powers, S., & Spitzer, A. (undated). *Clinical teaching behaviors that enhance the student's self-confidence as a nurse.* Unpublished.

ADDITIONAL READINGS

Brookfield, S. D. (1986). *Understanding and facilitating adult learning.* San Francisco: Jossey-Bass.

Infante, M. S. (1985). *The clinical laboratory in nursing education.* New York: Wiley.

Knowles, M. (1976). *The adult learner: A neglected species.* Houston: Gulf.

Knowles, M. S., & Associates. (1984). *Andragogy in action: Applying modern principles of adult learning.* San Francisco: Jossey-Bass.

Reilly, D. E., & Oermann, M. H. (1985). *The clinical field: Its use in nursing education.* Norwalk, CT: Appleton-Century-Crofts.

Schein, E. H. (1972). *Professional education: Some new directions.* New York: McGraw-Hill.

6

Expert Clinical Teaching

Barbara A. Hedin, PhD, RN

If this chapter had a subtitle, either "Knowing When to Let Them Fly" or "Making Sense Through Metaphors" would be strong contenders for the slot. The first phrase highlights the essence of the content being presented, and the latter, the means through which it is being described.

Initially this chapter presents a description of expert clinical teaching in the words of the practitioners themselves. Later it offers a brief overview of the research and writing that has been done in the area of clinical teaching. These two sections encourage the reader to discuss, reflect upon, and critique his or her own teaching practice. The third section takes a step back from the interviews and the literature and attempts to place them both in the broader framework of a critical theoretical perspective as a means of viewing and making sense of nursing curriculum and clinical teaching.

As we begin, let us turn to the function that metaphors can serve in accomplishing this task. In the words of Neil Postman,

> There is no test, textbook, syllabus, or lesson plan that any of us creates that does not reflect our preference for some metaphor of the mind, or of knowledge, or of the process of learning. Do you believe a student's mind to be a muscle that must be exercised? Or a garden that must be cultivated? Or a dark cavern that must be illuminated? Or an empty vessel that must be filled to overflowing? Whichever you favor, your metaphor will control—often without your being aware of it— how you will proceed as a teacher . . . All forms of discourse are metaphor-laden, and unless our students are aware of how metaphors shape arguments, organize perceptions, and control feelings, their understanding is severely limited (1988, pp. 29–30).

It is clear also that our understandings of our teaching practice are constrained as well is we fail to attend to the metaphors that guide our practice. Let us begin our dialogue on expert clinical teaching by looking at the metaphors that several nurse educators used to describe their practice.

INTERVIEWS WITH EXPERT CLINICAL FACULTY

Metaphors

When asked about their clinical teaching practice, nurse faculty used several different metaphors to capture the essence of their work. One educator used architecture, saying

> I used to say to the students: you are intent on laying bricks. Getting the mortar in and making it line up with the next brick. The junior students are building walls. They're building lots of walls and rooms. The senior students are building a building. A masters clinical specialist, a cathedral. But the person laying the bricks is also building a cathedral. It's all in your perspective. We lay the bricks together and we're asking them to see the cathedral.

Another nurse educator likened the importance of the relationship of the clinical faculty member to the student to the bond that is established "as if they have gone through the fire together."

Flying was a metaphor that was used by more than one individual.

> You've got to let them fly when they're ready to fly and not one minute before. So you have to know when, [and to do that] you've got to be right at the bedside.

> Once I had more experience [teaching] and had a clearer idea of what I could expect at the various levels, then I was able to go forward with that and be a little more risk taking as far as being able to pick out which students were able to handle one level and let them fly versus the ones that had to be kind of hand held for a little bit and helped to grow in a different way.

Gardening was described in quite some detail.

> I'm a gardener. Plant the seeds, provide the sunny environment, one that fosters growth, that's trust, that's confidence, supply for the student the confidence in herself that she lacks, to help her see her own proficiency as she moves along, so that she can develop a confidence base that can stand on some firm ground and ask questions about the muck ahead, and take that step with some degree of "Well, I did this, maybe I can do that." The plant grows from the inside. I don't understand what makes it grow . . . and flower. . . . All you can do is provide the environment in

which that can happen. A teaching environment that's safe for the student, approving, rewarding, reinforcing and rigorous in terms of expecting that they know what they're doing and holding to that—more as an ideal than as a punishment or a putdown. Magically, in spite of everything we do to help them, they'll grow. Pruning is required, and weeding is required, watering is required, and a lot of sunshine is required. It's amazing what people will do with that kind of an atmosphere.

Music was also offered as metaphor:

You try to look for more than the notes; you try to look for essentially the whole symphony, the whole piece of music. If you're teaching a student to play piano, and there are certain arpeggios, movements in that piece that are problematic, you may stress those and go over and over them. The student is learning and there will be mistakes; at some point they're competent in that piece of the task, but that's not enough because they still can't play the piece; then you move on to something else, maybe phrasing or mood or something. The full artistry of nursing, if ever achieved, is achieved some time after graduation. But at this student level, you are looking for putting together a synthesis of the pieces by caring for a patient, not doing a sterile dressing, not doing suctioning, but taking care of the whole patient. It's not realistic to expect that a student will do all that, anymore than you expect a piano student after four years of piano to sit down and do Van Cliburn. That's not the level that you expect, but there is a sort of sense of when they are putting it together enough; that they're not seeing pieces of the patient, they're not leaving out things . . . And the ability to discuss it and weave back and forth between the theoretical underpinnings and what they're doing. That's alot.

Music and flying were interwoven in one description.

Are we looking at a phenomenon that defies analysis to some degree? I know that's heretical, but we're talking about an interpersonal process that has all kinds of nuances that are unique to each nurse-client interaction. That calls for the nurse to play a new song on every trip on stage. What do you look for then? Certainly not the song that she's playing now, but her ability to transpose? How do you measure that? . . . We've got to show a student how to do aseptic procedure, [etc.] The student who can't play C is not going to play music as well as a student who can play C, and F, and B, and G. But that's not all of it. If they don't do that, they can't do this, but at what point do they fly?

Overview of the Interview Process

The data presented in this chapter were collected as part of a pilot study exploring expert practice in clinical teaching. The sample was obtained by requesting names of faculty members (who were identified as expert clinical nurse educators) from chairs and deans of nursing education programs. The interviews were semi-structured and began with discussion of a description of a clinical encounter which was defined as: "an interaction that you have had in which you feel your teaching made a difference in student learning."[1] The data are grouped into the areas of metaphors for clinical teaching, stated goals/aims of clinical teaching, attributes of faculty members, and the teaching role.

These categories are not exhaustive of all of those emerging from the data analysis, and neither is any one category fully explicated in this chapter. Rather, I have attempted to offer enough detail in the selected areas to convey the flavor of what was said, thereby the reader can gain some insight into the clinical teaching practice of expert nurse educators and enter into his or her own dialogue with the thoughts expressed. With this in mind, let us turn to the goals/aims that these nurse educators identified as giving direction to their clinical teaching.

Goals/Aims of Clinical Teaching

The categories for goals/aims fell into three broad areas: patient care, connecting/fitting, and questioning/judgment skills.

> The primary goal of clinical teaching, the *raison d'etre,* is patient care. Students are there to make sure the patients are taken care of.
>
> The important thing is to make sure that patient safety is maintained. Safety is the bottom line.
>
> It's making sure the patient gets taken care of and that students feel good about themselves.
>
> The goal of clinical teaching is facilitating their [the students'] fit. It is enabling their connecting: with themselves, the patients, the unit, etc.
>
> What I think is real important for students in the clinical area is to enjoy what they are doing, especially in baccalaureate programs. They spend so much time in class, they know how they're going to feel in the clinical area. This is what they have chosen to do and they go to the clinical area and they are so anxious they can never enjoy it; they can never connect with the people. Then something's wrong.
>
> If I can help reduce their anxiety enough so that they can sort of feed themselves, so that they can make some people connections, and then also work at developing their nursing practice however they're going to define that, then they can feel some success.
>
> If they can fall in love with themselves, with their own proficiency, with their own skill, they'll fall in love with nursing, and you'll have a lifelong learner.

---

[1] Adapted from P. Benner's (1984) work in the area of expert nursing practice, *From Novice to Expert: Excellence and Power in Clinical Nursing Practice.*

I think that was one of my [goals]; I tried very hard to keep in mind what it was going to be like for these women and young men when they got out of school, cause it's not the same as being a student.

That students know resources for learning and maximize their own ability to ask themselves questions and find answers to them. The more I look at it, the more I realize that the essence of education is what question does the student ask.

My goal wasn't to give them all the information, it was to teach them how to think about the situation and figure it out for themselves.

Faculty Attributes

Faculty were not asked to describe themselves nor what characteristics they thought they possessed. Rather, this information emerged from the interview data itself as faculty described their teaching practice. The data are grouped in six general categories: knowledge of self, shares self as a human being, reflective of clinical and teaching practice, characteristics, attitudes toward students, and clinical expertise.

Faculty revealed a high level of **self-knowledge** in their discussion of their practice. Statements such as "My choice to work in an acute environment tells me I like not quite being sure where the day is going to go . . . I like tension and anxiety"; "I know what works with me"; and "I may not be the best, but I'm alright" all show assessment of and reflection on their own likes and dislikes and strengths and limitations. This extended to an awareness of their effect on other people: "That was a lesson to me too. Heisenberg, the more you observe, the more you change what you observe. The closer you get into the picture, the more you disrupt the clinical experience and what's going on."

The clear intentionality on the part of the faculty **to share themselves as human beings** was a strong force in their teaching. They were committed to the importance of showing that they were human, made mistakes, and second-guessed themselves in situations. One instructor responded, "It's OK to be scared. See, I am too" and "Like in a crash or a code (or afterwards)—I didn't hesitate to show them my hands shaking, or say, 'Boy, that was really hairy.' They need to see that otherwise they're going to feel like they're abnormal." Faculty also sought to do this through sharing their own experiences as both student and nurse to help put students at ease.

An additional quality of these faculty was their **reflectiveness on their clinical and teaching practice.** They were engaged in constant self-appraisal in the clinical area and used such phrases as "My question to me was, 'Why couldn't I be more effective with her?'"

Characteristics of faculty included many that have been identified elsewhere in the nursing literature: a sense of humor ("You need to be able to cry with them [patients] and laugh with them too"), empathy, honesty, directness, openness, and taking a holistic view of the learner.

Faculty **attitudes toward learners** were characterized by a deep respect for them as human beings and a concerted effort to deal with them at their level of understanding. This included behaviors such as taking students aside to correct or criticize them; showing sensitivity when correcting mistakes; and relating to them with an awareness of their learning needs and knowledge base. It involved seeking to deal with students' perceptions of what was important to learn, which comes from their image of nursing. There was an attempt made at all times to treat learners as human beings and not just students ("I knew there were other things going on with her personally"). Concern and caring were earmarks of this relationship ("You matter to me") as was a commitment to the students and their future ("What will it be like for them?"). Trust was conveyed ("I know you can do it") as well as confidence in the learners (*allowing* them to feel confident). Faculty paid attention to the learners and sought to be fully accessible to them ("I am here for you").

Faculty were not asked about their own **clinical expertise** or whether they were engaged in ongoing clinical practice, but this subject arose in every interview, and in every case faculty were either actively engaged in practice or felt competent in practice as a result of immediate, prior nursing experience. They described themselves as being "in up to their elbows" and "in the middle of it all" in the clinical area with students, as the following descriptions clearly reveal. One faculty member shared this experience.

> I would not have grown if I had not taken care of that 19-year-old girl. I learned alot. I still learn alot from my practice. It gives me credibility. It gives me an idea of what's reasonable to expect . . . I'm not afraid to assign sick patients to my students because I know what's involved in their care. . . . The bell-wether is, "Can I take care of this patient?" If the answer is no, you shouldn't be assigning that patient.

In another instance this same nurse educator reflected on the relationship between courage and nursing practice.

> I have to have the courage to let them take care of a patient whose care is complex, who is hanging in an unstable condition where nursing care makes a significant difference minute by minute. I can't let them do that unless I know how it is doable, so that if they run into a problem, I know what we do next. . . . What [a faculty member] sets up, depends on what she feels comfortable with. That's a hard question that faculty don't look at too much. We need to look at it.

Another nurse faculty member said,

> It was both close contact with their patients and demonstration because I really was very actively involved with their patient care. I was not a

faculty member that sat in a conference room and had the students come with me, to me, to discuss their patients. I was out on the ward with the students because I typically assigned them to the most complicated and difficult patients on the ward, and felt like they needed some, not necessarily close supervision, but somebody that they could count on to be there and interactions with the patients were very important to me and I felt like they needed to see what it was like to be a grown-up taking care of patients and [to see] somebody with some experience doing it.

Faculty Roles

While faculty saw themselves fulfilling a number of different roles, those most commonly identified were the roles of facilitator of learning and modeler of nurse behaviors. Additional roles which were described, but will not be reviewed in detail here, include resource person, limit and standard setter, and evaluator. Under the role as facilitator of learning, the majority of behaviors described fell into the area of creating a safe space—physically and psychologically—for learning. This included providing learners the space and freedom to enjoy what they were doing,

> I just wanted [the students] to know that its a good job and it can be fun and real rewarding and they can't learn that if they're worried about whose going to come behind them and smack them down. They just can't do it.

providing positive feedback,

> That's the one thing when I went into teaching I wanted to make sure happened. When I was an undergraduate student, I felt that all week all I heard was negative things . . . because you can't do everything perfectly. . . . When I graduated from nursing school I had a bad feeling about myself. . . . I wanted to make sure they felt like they were doing a good job.

creating an atmosphere/environment of trust and open communication,

> I talk openly that what I want is open communication between us and that with us we're trying to forget the way things have been in other clinical areas, but this is the way it's going to be; when we get there I'm not aware of breaking that trust with them. But they don't quite know. It's not really been tested, so I try to give them as much freedom as I feel I safely can. I make sure that they know what's going on with their patients, what the plan of care is for today. . . . I try not to stand there and watch them. I have to tell them and then they have to see it. Words and behavior must be consistent.

and trying to get students beyond their anxiety:

> I worked with her alot one-on-one throughout the day and she never made any real connection with the patient. She never was able to get beyond her own anxiety.

One educator summed her thoughts up as follows:

> There are people who facilitate well and people who don't facilitate well. I think that's about all you can say. Because you can't get inside and what goes on inside is the learning. All teaching is ultimately self-teaching and nothing will be learned that is not self-taught. All you can really do is show vistas, entice, reward for stepping out, invite, and that sort of thing. But you can't punish, or push or shove anybody to learn anything anywhere.

In the realm of their roles as modelers of nurse behaviors, there were two aspects that faculty addressed. One was as model for the students to observe interacting with patients; and the second was in the student–faculty relationship which they felt should model the behaviors expected in nurse-patient interactions.

> I try to interact with the patient when I'm in there. I'm not just listening to what the student's saying, but they also compare themselves to me and to the nurses they see practicing around them.

> How do you teach anybody how to interact with a client if not by doing?

> I just feel like I'm not that different from the average learner and some of the skills are real complicated, even some of the interpersonal skills, and I just felt like they could do alot of their own thing, but they could also benefit from seeing me plus when you show them that you know how to do it, they listen to you when you tell them where they need to grow.

> Yet, we tell students to validate info with clients, confirm your impressions with them, and we turn around and evaluate students without validating our interpretations of what is happening. To what extent do we mete out to our clients, to our employees, to our subordinates, to our students, the kind of humanistic interaction that we demand of the nursing model nurse–client interaction?

> Faculty need to model the values and behaviors that we want students to exhibit in their own practice, and we need to use these in our relations with students.

While the value of faculty's personal reflections cannot be ignored, much of the data from the research studies which follow are derived from students' opinions on clinical teaching. Let us see what light they have shed on this topic.

THE LITERATURE ON CLINICAL TEACHING

My purpose is not to offer a comprehensive review of the literature on clinical teaching in nursing education but, rather, a more selective overview. The reader is encouraged to examine the various studies cited and draw his or her own conclusions.

Beginning with the oft quoted works of Barham (1965) and Jacobson (1966) on the effectiveness of teaching behaviors, much of the work that has been done in nursing since that time has continued to be primarily concerned with effective and ineffective teaching behaviors. Teacher characteristics have been identified (Armington, Reinikka, & Creighton, 1972; Brown, 1981; Mogan & Knox, 1987), as well as effective and ineffective teaching behaviors (Jacobson, 1966; Layton, 1969; Stafford, 1979; O'Shea & Parsons, 1979; Knox & Mogan, 1985), and comparisons of the relative importance assigned to behaviors by students and faculty (O'Shea & Parsons, 1979; Pugh, 1980; Brown, 1981; Knox & Mogan, 1985; Mogan & Knox, 1987). Research has been done using both the critical incident technique—or a modification thereof—(Barham, 1965; Jacobson, 1966; Wong, 1978; O'Shea & Parsons, 1979) as well as survey techniques drawing on categories of behaviors from earlier studies (Stafford, 1979; Pugh, 1980; Brown, 1981; Mogan & Knox, 1987), and observation and interview methods (Glass, 1971). In almost all studies, students have been used, and often, faculty along with students (Stafford, 1979; O'Shea & Parsons, 1979; Pugh, 1980; Brown, 1981; Mogan & Knox, 1987). The premise has been that the students, who are receiving the instruction, are the best judges of what effective teaching behaviors are.

In the majority of studies, the recommendation has been made that graduate schools should include this information in the education of future nurse educators or in faculty development programs (Jacobson, 1966; Wong, 1978; Pugh, 1980; Brown, 1981). It was also frequently suggested that further research is needed in this area and that the development of tools for measurement is needed (Wong, 1978; Knox & Mogan, 1985; Zimmerman & Waltman, 1986; Windsor, 1987). Pugh (1986) noted that much of the work seemed disjointed and did not build upon previous studies. As a result, new lists of behaviors were reinvented and while similar to previous one, they did not relate closely enough to allow for comparisons across studies. A number of authors have raised the significant issue of the discrepancy between faculty knowing what to do and actually doing it in terms of the utilization of ideal clinical teaching behaviors (Pugh, 1980; Meleca, Schimpfhauser, Witteman, & Sachs, 1981; Infante, 1985; McCabe, 1985).

Noting which of the effective clinical behaviors appeared consistently is quite useful. Zimmerman and Waltman, in their 1986 review of the literature on these behaviors noted that many of the behaviors identified in the various studies they reviewed were mentioned in Jacobson's earlier study.

Jacobson (1966) used a modified form of the critical incident technique in which students were asked to describe in writing as many recent effective and ineffective incidents as possible in a 50-minute time span. A total of 1,182 usable incidents were obtained from 961 undergraduate students in 5 university schools of nursing. Fifty-eight critical requirements for the teaching of nursing were derived from these incidents, which were then grouped into 6 general categories: availability to students, general knowledge and professional competence, interpersonal relations with students and others, teaching practices, personal characteristics, and evaluation practices. Exemplary behaviors found in these categories included:

1. Keeps self available to students in stressful situations and as a resource person.
2. Demonstrates own ability as a nurse and teacher by identifying principles basic to practice, planning for depth and continuity of care, making students aware of professional responsibility, etc.
3. Shows skill in interpersonal relationships by alleviating student anxieties, conveying confidence in and respect for the student, correcting student tactfully without devaluating the student, etc.
4. Teaching practices include having a sense of timing, knowing when student is ready to proceed, reviewing plan of action with student and then letting student go ahead, planning experiences for students when new and unexpected learning situations occur, etc.
5. Personal characteristics include showing warmth, sympathy, and human emotions; being honest and direct with students; maintaining an interest and enthusiasm that is "catching"; etc.
6. Evaluation practices include being fair in evaluations, telling student she has done well; being concerned with learning rather than testing; etc.

A number of the studies generated a list of behaviors that were categorized as effective or ineffective, without placing these behaviors in the wider context of teaching in the clinical arena, and more specifically, without addressing the aims/purposes/goals of clinical teaching. Without this broader discussion, the danger exists of manufacturing lists of behaviors to be imitated in an instrumental means/ends rationale. We should especially consider others areas that emerged in the interviews previously discussed that were critical attributes of expert clinical faculty—such as self-knowledge and reflection on one's teaching and nursing practice—that do not come to light through research methodologies that only focus on what occurs in the teacher–student interaction.

A FRAMEWORK FOR A CRITICAL PERSPECTIVE ON CLINICAL TEACHING

This section of the chapter draws most heavily on the work of Jurgen Habermas (1970; 1971; 1979) and Shirley Grundy (1987). Habermas is a German critical theorist known for his prolific writings over the past three decades in the area of social philosophy. Grundy has applied Habermas' work, and especially the conceptualization of knowledge constitutive interests, to curriculum development in her book, *Curriculum: Product or praxis.*

Knowledge Constitutive Interests

According to Habermas, there are certain fundamental orientations of the human species in which knowledge and action can be grounded. He identifies these interests as the technical interest, the practical interest, and the emancipatory interest (Habermas, 1970). These are referred to as knowledge constitutive interests. The use of the word interest connotes the aim of understanding one's guiding motive and the intentions behind the act that shape one's actions and behaviors. To speak of these knowledge constitutive interests is to address the way and the wherefore in which we operate in the world and carry out our work of seeking knowledge, doing research, interacting, and teaching nursing. These three interests can be used as a lens to organize and make sense of our actions and behaviors.

Action carried out in a technical interest is concerned with control and management of one's surroundings: the environment, people, etc. It is characterized by a means/end rationality or instrumental reasoning—"the ends justify the means" kind of thinking and acting. The emphasis is on the outcome rather than the process.

Action undertaken in a practical interest is concerned with self and mutual understanding and intersubjective meaning. Because it is concerned with the notion of surviving along with, a moral component is introduced in which action "for the good" is sought. One seeks to understand the environment in order to interact with it, rather than to have control over it. Understanding and the making of meaning are chief elements of the practical interest.

Action and behavior carried on within an emancipatory interest is concerned with the identification and elimination of constraints—outmoded structures and relations—that impede open discourse, and autonomous and responsible action. It is concerned with the empowerment of individuals as autonomous and responsible agents in the world.

Curriculum as Product, Practice, and Praxis

Curriculum as Product. Curriculum developed within a technical interest is identified by Grundy as product-oriented. Curriculum makers have the idea—or ideal—of something, and work toward that as the end sought. The type of action employed can be referred to as "making" action, product-oriented. The student is the product. The teacher uses skills to reproduce students into an idea that already exists. There is a hierarchy of theory and practice. Power relations in this situation are characterized by control being in the hands of the faculty, who control the learner and the learning environment. "[The] fundamental interest [is] in controlling the educational environment so that an educational product may result which accords with certain prespecified objectives" (Grundy, 1987, p. 31). Knowledge is often perceived of and presented as sets of rules or procedures or unquestioned truths.

Curriculum as Practice. Curriculum development within a practical interest is concerned with making meaning through interpretation which calls for human judgment. It is not a matter of looking to a set of rules or preconceived ideas of what should be as the basis for action and imposing these no matter what, but, rather, making decisions about the meaning of the rules and situations in which they are to be applied before action is taken. Knowledge is made personal by experience and reasoning. There is a "fitting on of knowledge" to the individual.

Action is carried out with regard to the human good; choice and deliberation are involved. There is concern with what is good, rather than necessarily correct. A particular result is not sought, but a state of being. Since practical action involves human interaction, the emphasis is on the importance of all participants in relationships as subjects and not objects.

At the heart of curriculum created in a practical interest is the development of meaning for the learner and the avoidance of imposing someone else's meaning on the learner. One is not satisfied with only cognitive justification for content, for example, but moral criteria for "the good" as well (Grundy, 1986). The resulting pedagogy is a situated one. It is situated or connected in the learner's reality and concerned with making meaning for the individual and group within that context.

Curriculum as Praxis. Emancipatory action, the knowledge orientation underlying the basis for action in developing a curriculum as praxis, develops out of a practical interest but is not an inevitable development or progression from it. If practical action situates pedagogy in the learner's reality, emancipatory action situates the educational interaction in its social context and illuminates the social construction of reality and hence, its ability to be transformed. Within such a perspective, the social world is posited as not being given or natural, as is a tree, for example. There are no universal, immutable laws governing functioning and relationships within the social education world. Hence, what we experience in educational systems is not the only world that could be, although it may reflect the dominant ideas of a culture.

As such, to view curriculum as praxis is to recognize that curricula are social constructions that have been created within a socially constrained world. The aim is not to attain to "the perfect curriculum" (since there isn't one), but, rather, to hold before us the creation of learning conditions and a learning environment that empowers individuals to participate in their reality—including public discourse—as autonomous and responsible agents. This means that an essential part of the education process is concerned with taking a critical, reflective view of the education process itself to identify and transform existing constraints to full participation of all individuals.

It is important to bear in mind throughout this discussion that the interests are not exclusive orientations, but rather, that one generally has a predominant mode in which he or she operates. The identification of one's metaphors may help one identify one's orientation.

An Illustration: Music as Metaphor

In order to elaborate on these ideas and the meaning and fruitfulness that they may hold for nursing, I will use the metaphor of teaching music and carry it through the three knowledge constitutive interests, briefly discussing assumptions, actions, means, and ends for each to highlight the differences among them.

The Technical Interest. To teach music within a technical interest, in which the curriculum is treated as a product, posits an underlying assumption that the teacher knows *the* song. The teacher's actions are directed toward teaching the students that song and the role of the teacher is that of information giver. The teacher's aim is to teach the students the notes, how to play them, and how to put them together into the song. He or she is concerned with finding the most effective and efficient means of teaching students the song. The end is that all the students learn *the* song.

The Practical Interest. Teaching music in the practical interest is based on the assumption that the teacher knows *a* song (which changes or is revised over time as he or she continues to grow and learn). The teacher's actions are geared toward teaching the students the notes that one uses in playing and composing songs and in seeking to facilitate the student's putting together the notes into their own songs. Their songs may be the same song as the teacher's, but may also be a transposition, use a different rhythm, or be an entirely different song. The teacher's attitude is one of "See, this is my song. What's yours?" The role of the teacher is that of (life-long) learner. The end is that the students learn *a* song, and the means are enacted in a situated pedagogy in which the lives and experiences of the learner are respected. There is a fit sought between that which is being taught and the personhood of the learner.

The Emancipatory Interest. Teaching music with an emancipatory interest as the orientation for action would mean seeking to situate one's action of teaching within the socially constructed world. Hence, one would be concerned with such issues as: In order for you to learn and play your song, and for me to play mine and teach you—what are the necessary conditions? What are the constraints that act on teacher–student relationships—in the classroom, in this institution, in this society? What counts for knowledge? And who decides? And so forth. The teacher's role is that of agent of empowerment, both for him or herself and for the students.

Clinical Teaching in Nursing: Where Are We?

While to categorize and label curricula as being developed and implemented from a technical interest, a practical interest, or an emancipatory interest may appear at first to be quite a different way of approaching the area of curriculum and clinical teaching within nursing, it is nonetheless very congruent with current streams of thinking in nursing, whose proponents may not necessarily use this terminology. One has only to look at the work of Bevis (1988) and Diekelmann (1988) to see the lines of convergence. Both of these nurse educators critique the exclusive use of Tyler's behaviorist model as the only legitimate curriculum model for nursing education, and offer alternative models for education into professional nursing practice. A close look at this discussion reveals that the Tyler curriculum model falls within "curriculum as product" ways of thinking—a technical interest—that was outlined earlier. I would also suggest that much of the research that has been done on clinical teaching which has focused on effective and ineffective teaching behaviors without discussion of the full context of learning, the aims sought, etc., also falls within this interest area.

On the other hand, the groundbreaking work of Bevis (1988) and Diekelmann (1988) in developing a "Professional or Educative Model" and a "Dialogue and Meaning Model" of curriculum, respectively, falls within the realm of curriculum as practice in which the pedagogy is situated in the learner's reality and a deep respect for the learner is evidenced. The interviews with expert clinical nursing faculty also indicate that their practice falls into this realm. The types of metaphors used and the ways in which they were described and puzzled over, their concern with self-knowledge and reflection on their practice, their deep respect for their learners as whole human beings, and their honoring of where they were are among the indicators which point to this.

To posit nursing curriculum as praxis would seem to require strong elements of a critical reflection on the educational moment in which one's teaching practice is placed within the social context and in which the role of nurses, role expectations, definitions, and the health care system, are critically examined. While I believe this is being done in the various instances discussed to varying degrees, it is not the predominant mode in which these activities are carried out.

CONCLUSION

We have explored the words, expressions, and metaphors that clinical faculty use to describe their practice; we have reviewed some of the research that has been done on effective and ineffective teaching behaviors; and we have discussed in broad strokes and with the use of metaphor, the use of the knowledge constitutive interests as a way to make sense of these areas. This leads to further questions rather than definitive answers, which somehow seems appropriate to our thinking in this developing area. Therefore I close by posing the following questions for the reader's continuing thought and reflection:

- What metaphors would you use to describe your teaching practice?
- Are your teaching practices congruent with the goals you hope to achieve?
- What facilitates your teaching?
- What is stopping you from teaching as you would prefer?
- Does the level of teaching (undergraduate, graduate) or the type of program (ADN, BSN, graduate) mandate the interest in which it is conducted? Are there qualitative differences among these or only quantitative?
- What does the nature of nursing demand of the education process of its practitioners?
- What are the constraints—both internal (personal) and external (classroom/institutional/societal)—to putting this educational process in place?

Our consciousness is the ceiling of our potential. It is through systematic study of and personal reflection on our teaching practices that we will be able to expand our consciousness to enable us to teach in ways that lead to transformation and learning for all participants.

REFERENCES

Armington, C., Reinikka, E. A., & Creighton, H. (1972). Student evaluation: Threat or incentive? *Nursing Outlook, 20*(12), 789–792.

Barham, V. Z. (1965). Identifying effective behaviors of the nursing instructor through critical incidents. *Nursing Research, 14,* 65–69.

Benner, P. (1984). *From novice to expert: Excellence and power in clinical nursing practice.* Menlo Park, CA: Addison-Wesley.

Bevis, E. O. (1988). New directions for a new age. In *Curriculum revolution: Mandate for change* (pp. 27–52). New York: National League for Nursing.

Brown, S. T. (1981). Faculty and student perceptions of effective clinical teachers. *Journal of Nursing Education, 20*(9), 4–15.

Diekelmann, N. (1988). Curriculum revolution: A theoretical and philosophical mandate for change. In *Curriculum revolution: Mandate for change* (pp. 137–157). New York: National League for Nursing.

Glass, H. P. (1971). *Teaching behavior in the nursing laboratory in selected baccalaureate nursing programs in Canada.* Doctoral dissertation, Teachers College, Columbia University.

Grundy, S. (1987). *Curriculum: Product or praxis.* London: Falmer Press.

Habermas, J. (1970). *Toward a rational society: Student protest, science and politics* (J. Shapiro, Trans.). Boston: Beacon Press. (Original work published 1968)

Habermas, J. (1971). *Knowledge and human interests* (J. Shapiro, Trans.). Boston: Beacon Press. (Original work published 1968)

Habermas, J. (1979). *Communication and the evolution of society* (T. McCarthy, Trans.). Boston: Beacon Press. (Original work published 1976)

Infante, M. S. (1985). *The clinical laboratory in nursing education* (2nd ed.). New York: Wiley.

Jacobson, M. D. (1966). Effective and ineffective behavior of teachers of nursing as determined by their students. *Nursing Research, 15*(3), 218–224.

Knox, J. E., & Mogan, J. (1985). Important clinical teacher behaviors as perceived by university nursing faculty, students and graduates. *Journal of Advanced Nursing, 10,* 25–30.

Layton, M. M. (1969). How instructors' attitudes affect students. *Nursing Outlook, 17,* 27–29.

McCabe, B. W. (1985). The improvement of instruction in the clinical area: A challenge waiting to be met. *Journal of Nursing Education, 24*(6), 255–257.

Meleca, C. B., Schimpfhauser, F., Witteman, J. K., & Sachs, L. (1981). Clinical instruction in nursing: A national survey. *Journal of Nursing Education, 20*(8), 32–40.

Mogan, J., & Knox, J. E. (1987). Characteristics of 'best' and 'worst' clinical teachers as perceived by university faculty and students. *Journal of Advanced Nursing, 12,* 331–337.

O'Shea, H. S., & Parsons, M. K. (1979). Clinical instruction: Effective and ineffective teachers behaviors. *Nursing Outlook, 27*(6), 411–415.

Postman, N. (1988). *Conscientious objections: Stirring up trouble about language, technology, and education.* New York: Knopf.

Pugh, E. J. (1980). Factors influencing congruence between beliefs, intentions, and behavior in the clinical teaching of nursing. Doctoral dissertation, Northwestern University. *Dissertation Abstracts International, 41*(6).

Pugh, E. J. (1986). Research on clinical teaching. In W. L. Holzemer (Ed.), *Review of research in nursing education* (Vol. 1, pp. 73–92). New York: National League for Nursing.

Stafford, L. F. (1979). Determining effective nursing teacher behaviors in clinical settings (Doctoral dissertation, Texas A&M University, 1978). *Dissertation Abstracts International, 39*(7), 4154A. Listed in *DAI* in 1979, dissertation completed in 1978.

Windsor, A. (1987). Nursing students perceptions of clinical experience. *Journal of Nursing Education, 26*(4), 150–154.

Wong, S. (1978). Nurse–teacher behaviors in the clinical field: Apparent effect on nursing students' learning. *Journal of Advanced Nursing, 3,* 369–372.

Zimmerman, L., & Waltman, N. (1986). Effective clinical behaviors of faculty: A review of the literature. *Nurse Educator, 11*(1), 31–34.

BIBLIOGRAPHY: CLINICAL TEACHING

Carpenito, L. J., & Duespohl, T. A. (1985). *A guide for effective clinical instruction* (2nd ed.). Rockville, MD: Aspen.

deTornyay, R. (1984). Research on the teaching–learning process in nursing education. In H. H. Werley & J. J. Fitzpatrick (Eds.), *Annual review of nursing research* (Vol. 2, pp. 193–210). New York: Springer Publishing.

deTornyay, R., & Thompson, M. A. (1987). *Strategies for teaching nursing* (3rd ed.). New York: Wiley.

Flagler, S., Loper-Powers, S., & Spitzer, A. (1988). Clinical teaching is more than evaluation alone! *Journal of Nursing Education, 27*(8), 342–348.

Hawkins, J. W. (1981). *Clinical experiences in collegiate nursing education: Selection of clinical agencies.* New York: Springer Publishing.

Henning, E. D. (1974). *Perceptions of clinical laboratory activities in baccalaureate programs in nursing.* Doctoral dissertation, Teachers College, Columbia University.

Infante, M. S. (1981). Toward effective and efficient use of the clinical laboratory. *Nurse Educator,* (Jan–Feb), 16–19.

Karns, P. J., & Schwab, T. A. (1982). Therapeutic communication and clinical instruction. *Nursing Outlook, 21*(1), 39–43.

Karuhije, H. F. (1986). Educational preparation for clinical teaching: Perceptions of the nurse educator. *Journal of Nursing Education, 25*(4), 137–144.

Kiker, M. (1973). Characteristics of the effective teacher. *Nursing Outlook, 21,* 721–723.

Mannion, M. (1968). *A taxonomy of instructional behaviors applicable to the guidance of learning activities in the clinical setting in baccalaureate nursing education.* Doctoral dissertation, The Catholic University of America.

Rauen, K. C. (1974). The clinical instructor as role model. *The Journal of Nursing Education, 13,* 33–40.

Reilly, D. E. (1978). *Teaching and evaluating the affective domain in nursing programs.* New Jersey: Charles B. Slack.

Schneider, H. L. (1979). *Evaluation of nursing competence.* Boston: Little, Brown, & Company.

Schweer, J. E., & Gebbie, K. M. (1976). *Creative teaching in clinical nursing.* St. Louis: Mosby.

Smith, D. W. (1968). *Perspectives on clinical teaching.* New York: Springer Publishing.

Stuebbe, B. (1981). Student and faculty perspectives on the role of nursing instructors. *Journal of Nursing Education, 7*(9), 4–9.

Van Hoozer, H. L., Bratton, B. D., Ostmoe, P. M., Weinholz, D., Craft, M. J., Gjerde, C. L., & Albanese, M. A. (1987). *The teaching process: Theory and practice in nursing.* Norwalk, CT: Appleton-Century-Crofts.

Van Ort, S. R., & Putt, A. M. (1985). *Teaching in collegiate schools of nursing.* Boston: Little, Brown, & Company.

Wang, A. M., & Blumberg, P. (1983). A study on interaction techniques of nursing faculty in the clinical area. *Journal of Nursing Education, 22*(4), 144–151.

Zimmerman, L., & Westfall, J. (1988). The development and validation of a scale measuring effective clinical teaching behaviors. *Journal of Nursing Education, 27*(6), 274–277.

BIBLIOGRAPHY: CRITICAL SOCIAL THEORY/NURSING

Allen, D. G. (1985). Nursing research and social control: Alternative models of science that emphasize understanding and emancipation. *Image, 17*(2), 58–64.

Allen, D. G. (1987). Critical social theory as a model for analyzing ethical issues in family and community health. *Family and Community Health, 10*(1), 63–72.

Allen, D., Benner, P., & Diekelmann, N. (1986). Three paradigms for nursing research: Methodological implications. In P. Chinn (Ed.), *Nursing research methodology: Issues and implementation* (pp. 23–38). Rockville, MD: Aspen.

Bullough, R. V., Goldstein, S. L., & Holt, L. (1984). *Human interests in the curriculum: Teaching and learning in a technological society.* New York: Teachers College Press.

Connerton, P. (Ed.). (1976). *Critical sociology: Selected readings.* New York: Penguin.

Geuss, R. (1981). *The idea of a critical theory: Habermas and the Frankfurt School.* Cambridge: Cambridge University Press.

Habermas, J. (1970). *Toward a rational society: Student protest, science and politics* (J. Shapiro, Trans.). Boston: Beacon Press. (Original work published 1968)

Habermas, J. (1971). *Knowledge and human interests* (J. Shapiro, Trans.). Boston: Beacon Press. (Original work published 1968)

Habermas, J. (1979). *Communication and the evolution of society* (T. McCarthy, Trans.). Boston: Beacon Press. (Original work published 1976)

Hedin, B. A. (1986). Nursing, education and emancipation: An application of the critical theoretical approach to nursing research. In P. Chinn (Ed.), *Nursing research methodology: Issues and implementation* (pp. 133–146). Rockville, MD: Aspen.

Held, D. (1980). *Introduction to critical social theory: Horkheimer to Habermas.* Berkeley: University of California Press.

Schroyer, T. (1973). *The critique of domination: The origins and development of critical theory.* Boston: Beacon Press.

Thompson, J. L. (1987). Critical scholarship: The critique of domination in nursing. *Advances in Nursing Science, 10*(1), 27–38.

7

Transforming Barriers in Nursing Education

Verle Waters, MA, RN

THE QUESTION OF EDUCATIONAL MOBILITY

Why is educational mobility in nursing still an issue which needs to be examined? Nurses have been writing and speechifying on this subject for 25 years, and can point to an extensive bibliography on educational and career mobility. Nonetheless, the course of nursing thought and action regarding educational mobility is uneven and puzzlingly inconsistent. Because educational mobility remains an issue despite the thought, time, effort, and paper devoted to it since the mid 1960s, one can only conclude that the barriers to mobility are not easily transformed. If they were, the problem would have been solved and we would not still be seeking answers to questions about educational mobility in nursing.

In a technical sense, we know the answers. There are articulated programs, career ladder programs, second step programs, upper two programs, upper one programs, external degree programs, and outreach programs. We have portfolio evaluations, standardized test evaluations, competency tests, and teacher-made tests. We have bridge courses, transition courses, and advanced placement. There are associate degree programs which admit only LPNs, and both baccalaureate and master's programs which admit only RNs. There are generic tracks, degree completion tracks, upgrade tracks, and fast tracks. There are many successful programs, admission and placement procedures, courses, and studies which show that RNs who become BSNs move into leadership positions, go on for graduate study, say they think more critically, and say they have more self-confidence (MacLean, Knoll, & Kinney, 1985).

Still, there is a problem. There are barriers to educational mobility, and in the light of what the future of nursing education holds, it is important that those barriers be transformed. What are the barriers to educational mobility in nursing, and why to they persist?

BACKGROUND

There are historical and ideological factors going back to the beginning of nursing in the United States that bring complexity and ambivalence into the educational mobility discussion. During the 1960s and early 1970s, the ambivalence was expressed in the inconsistency between the decisive position of the National League for Nursing (NLN) regarding the definition of the basic baccalaureate generalist program, and the expression of support by NLN for what was called the open curriculum.

Educational mobility was a lively topic in NLN circles at that time. Strong beliefs about what liberal education represented in the program of study for a nurse supported strong positions on curriculum requirements. Boyle, Ren, and Paterson stated in their 1962 article that ". . . liberal education precedes and is basic to professional education . . ." Kibrick (1968) echoed this, saying that:

> Nursing practice in collegiate programs builds on and integrates the liberal arts into the nursing curriculum; to give college credit for nursing courses taken apart from the liberal arts or before acquiring a broad base in the arts and sciences would contradict the entire philosophy and practice of collegiate education.

The *Statement of Beliefs* from the National League for Nursing Board of Directors (1964) called for the end of special programs for RNs, and put forth the notion that there was one baccalaureate program, the generic program, which RNs along with other students would have to complete. This implied that not only would there be just one baccalaureate curriculum, but also by definition professional nursing could be taught only on a base of liberal education. For RNs, particularly diploma graduates, the consequence was that obtaining a bachelor's degree in nursing required a minimum of four full years of study, with participation in all nursing courses. The reasoning was that these nursing courses would be different from any the nurse had taken in a diploma program, by virtue of the fact that liberal arts study had preceded them. Not every diploma graduate who went into BS programs at that time agreed, and, not surprisingly, a counter movement took shape in the mid 1970s. Sonoma State University (1974) for example, proposed that

> We believe that associate degree or equivalent nursing preparation can be an integral part of and does form the foundation upon which professional nursing can be built.

CURRICULUM IN CONFLICT

Most nurses working in nursing education during the 1970s were aware that it was a period of lively discourse on the topic of educational mobility, with many meetings and articles devoted to airing of the pros and cons of what was called, as an umbrella term, "the open curriculum." Surfacing in the opposition to this "open curriculum" and bolstering the arguments for preserving the ideals of the baccalaureate curriculum was an old concern which plagues our thinking still today: a long-standing feeling of uncertainty about the educational qualifications of those educated in a program which is "less than" whatever program it is that we are teaching in. Susan Reverby (1987) has pointed out nursing's historic animus toward the lesser trained nurse. Speaking of nursing's effort around the turn of the century to strengthen its professional strength and visibility, Reverby writes:

> In organizing professional nursing associations, they sought, through voluntary and legislative means, to limit the numbers in nursing and to standardize and raise its educational requirements . . . In doing so, they attacked the background, training, and ideology of most of working nurses. (p. 121)

This concern for the educational quality of shorter programs and the effect on professionalism has been expressed in many ways by different speakers. Anderson (1972) questioned: "What would be the consequences of planning the bachelor's on the base of an associate degree in nursing? Inevitably, the bachelor's curriculum would be diluted and then the base for graduate education weakened." This sense that the lesser trained nurse has an almost unredeemable deficit by virtue of her educational background manifests itself in various barriers and problems today. We may label the LPNs and RNs who present themselves to enter our programs in negative terms, and speak of them as having "LPN (or RN) mentality"; we find them difficult to socialize. We are burdened by mixed and conflicting values. On the one hand, we embrace egalitarian, democratic values in our profession. Nurses are a group with many members who have been educationally mobile, have moved up the ladder, and are proud of it. We respond to the AMA and its RCT proposal by saying we already have the levels the AMA is proposing, *and,* we point out, they are not dead ends. On the other hand, there is a lasting and strong ethos that we must not embrace nursing as a multilevel, pluralistic, rationally connected system. There is the belief that to sanction defined relationships between educational levels would be academically and professionally shoddy. Perhaps the best observation on our conflicted ideology was made by Ruth Matheney (1975): "Many nursing educators still think that, if nurses graduate from a 'terminal' program, they should at least have the good grace to remain terminal" (p. 85).

BREAKING THE BARRIERS

Many barriers have tumbled in the years since the open curriculum initiatives of the 1970s. New opportunities have been created for nurses who want to further their education, and a variety of excellent procedures and programs encourage and support educational mobility. Nonetheless, there is institutional and regional unevenness. A recent study in California revealed a surprising amount of variation in curriculum practices which can facilitate or hinder educational mobility. A survey of the 70 associate degree programs in the state revealed that total required units (credit hours) for graduation from an ADN program ranged from 62 to 115, and for graduation from a BSN (generic) program the range was from 123 to 144. Table 1 shows selected results of the surveys.

The survey of the baccalaureate programs also asked for the maximum possible number of units (credit hours) that an RN who graduated from an associate degree program can transfer and apply toward graduation requirements in the BSN program. The variation found within one state, within one educational system (the public state university system) came as a surprise. Students are permitted, depending on the baccalaureate program in California they choose, to transfer as few as 2 or as many as 36 course units (credits), with the average being 26 (Hansen, 1988).

Unquestionably, institutional policies and conventions limit articulation possibilities. Upper-division vis-à-vis lower-division distinctions create barriers in many institutions. Still, some nursing programs seem to find creative ways for transforming barriers. In higher education outside of nursing, upper-division credit is frequently awarded without controversy for previous lower-division study. Nursing hold strong, but not uniform, values and beliefs in this area; one faculty will feel comfortable with practices that another finds unsound. Nursing's value orientation is diametrical. At one pole, we believe in an essentially pragmatic position and

TABLE 1. Semester Units Required for Degree in Nursing California Associate and Baccalaureate Programs

	ASSOCIATE DEGREE (N = 56)		BACCALAUREATE DEGREE (N = 18)	
	Median	Range	Median	Range
Total Units	76	62–115	130	123–144
Nursing Units	41	36–74	60	50–68
General Ed Units	35	21–54	69	53–90

at the other, an essentially ideologic position—which gives rise to mixed and erroneous perceptions that constitute barriers. We need to recognize and correct the misperceptions which inhibit educational mobility.

NLN accreditation criteria are said to be a barrier to articulation. Although cited frequently, it is a myth that specific admission practices are either prohibited or allowed in accreditation criteria. The perception that there is no difference between AD and BS in the nursing educational program constitutes another barrier. Some ADN educators debunk upper-division nursing in a professional program as "no different," citing an equal number of class hours in an ADN program, common texts, or other similar educational practices. It is the joint responsibility of ADN and BSN educators to identify (or create) the differences as well as identifying similarities, so that students who receive both an ADN and a BSN education benefit from the best of both. The attitudes carried by the students themselves frequently constitute a barrier. The student perception that there is "always" duplication of nursing knowledge and experience when they return to school inhibits articulation success. On the other hand, if a strong case that the required upper-division nursing courses are different from the ADN or diploma nursing courses cannot be made, a barrier exists. Institutional constraints, perceptions, and attitudes can and do function as barriers to educational mobility.

The role of demographic factors in educational mobility within nursing may ultimately be the compelling rationale that transforms all barriers and brings about a predictable educational system. Demographics, interestingly enough, has now been added as a newcomer to the list of social sciences. It is said that of all the social sciences, demographics is most like the science of celestial mechanics—we look for the higher unseen engines that make the social system work in certain ways. There is a huge unseen engine—the population of students who will be in our nursing pipeline—which argues for predictability in educational mobility.

A 1985 report by Harold L. Hodgkinson spells out the demographics of education from kindergarten through graduate school. He challenges our tendency to look only at our own institutional segment, whether community college, college, or university, and to see our own educational enterprise as a discrete and separate unit shaped by unique factors and forces. In fact, Hodgkinson points out, education from kindergarten through graduate school is *All One System,* the title of his study. The stream of people who are moving through at any one time make it a system and ultimately define what it is and what it is doing. He cautions all of us in education to observe the major changes occurring in birth and immigrant groups that are now shaping and will continue to dramatically shape the educational enterprise. Hodgkinson cites these data:

1. There are substantial increases in the number of children entering the school system with backgrounds that predict major learning

difficulties. These include, first, the rapidly increasing numbers of children born out of marriage to teenage mothers. Hodgkinson states that about 700,000 of the annual 3.3 million births in the United States are almost assured of being either educationally retarded or "difficult to teach." (He cites correlations between prematurity and low birth weight, and learning disabilities.) Secondly, he reminds us that children born into poverty enter school with backgrounds associated with learning difficulty, and that the number of such children is increasing. A child under 6 today is 6 times more likely to be poor than a person over 65.

2. Asian-Americans represent 44 percent of all immigrants admitted to the United States. Asian-American youths are heavily involved in public schools; a high percentage graduate and attend college. They present a particular challenge in higher education because of their understandable difficulty in verbal tasks, yet higher than average scores in mathematical ability measures.

3. By approximately the year 2000, America will be a nation in which one out of every three people will be nonwhite. At this point minorities will cover a broader socioeconomic range than ever before, making simplistic treatment of their needs even less useful.

4. There is, and will continue to be, an absolute decline in the number of 18-to 24-year-olds. In addition, high school retention rates are decreasing: 14% of white students are dropping out, 20% of black students, and 30% of Hispanic. Concurrently, there is an increase in the number of high school dropouts who acquire the General Equivalency Diploma, then apply to a college or university that will accept them. Hodgkinson summarizes the challenge to higher education in these words:

> The rapid increase in minorities among the youth population is here to stay. We need to make a major commitment, as educators, to see that all our students in higher education have the opportunity to perform academically at a high level. There will be barriers of color, language, culture, attitude that will be greater than any we have faced before, as Spanish-speaking students are joined by those from Thailand and Vietnam. The task will be not to lower the standards, but to increase the effort. For the next 15 years at least, we will have to work harder with the limited number of young people we have to work with.

Although the 18-to 24-year-old group will decline in size until 1994, there is another group available to bolster sagging college enrollments. The "baby boomers" are now in the peak middle years of earning and learning; they are the possible growth component in postsecondary education. There will be constant expansion of the world population until this group begins to retire in the year 2000!

The Education Commission of the States made recommendations to state leaders for "transforming the state role in undergraduate education." Eight challenges facing undergraduate education are listed, among them: "To meet the educational needs of an increasingly diverse student population. Of the 12 million students enrolled in our 3,300 colleges and universities, only 2 million attend full time, live on campus, and are 18–22 years old. By 1992 half of all college students will be more than 25 years old, and 20 percent will be more than 35" (pp. 14–15).

The demography, that huge unseen engine that ultimately drives the system, foretells a continuing stream of students entering the several levels of our pluralistic nursing educational system. The unprecedented diversity of students argues for a system wherein people can begin study at many different levels of academic achievement and obtain the remedial, academic, and financial assistance that will allow them to succeed. Education needs to be available in negotiable units of time and in a manageable location. There is need for articulation between segments that allow the adult learner to enter, leave, and reenter, building educational increments toward the individual's highest level of achievement, limited only by ability and personal choice.

The arresting message in the Hodgkinson monograph is in the title: *All One System.* More important than the profile of the student population is the principal idea: the segments of the educational enterprise are not separate entities, but are bound one to another by what they hold in common and ineluctably share—namely—the students. Hodgkinson states that hard as it is to believe, graduate students were at one time third-graders; so, too, in our smaller universe. Nursing graduate students were once in associate degree, diploma, or bachelor's degree programs; increasingly, baccalaureate students were once AD or diploma students. Baccalaureate program faculty are experiencing a very rapid change in the student population. In 1975, 10 percent of students in BSN programs were RNs. That grew to 30 percent in 1985. The trend suggests that by 1990, 50 percent of students in BSN programs will be graduates of ADN or diploma programs.

Nursing's history and past practices in providing educational mobility show a strong reluctance to embrace the pluralistic multilevel education system in nursing. Frequently, the ideas about educational mobility (i.e., encouraging LPNs to apply to ADN programs and RNs to BSN programs) are couched in terms of an all-out short-term remedial effort until the system can be changed in more permanent ways—eliminating LPN programs, phasing out diploma, or gearing up for the education of all RNs in baccalaureate programs. In that view, educational mobility is needed as a temporary measure to move from *now* to *then.* Such a position ignores the future as it already exists and is moving inexorably toward us while overlooking the basic truth that it is the students who determine the educational system.

Providing educational mobility does not require standardization of the educational system itself. The desired goal is not uniformity, rather it is predictability. A multilevel system with options, alternatives, ladders, crossovers, entrances and exits, internal and external degrees, and more is not necessarily a system in disarray; it may be enlightened, orderly, logical, sensitive, rich in diversity and the opportunities it offers, and effective in the essential social service it provides.

TOWARD THE FUTURE OF EDUCATIONAL MOBILITY

Transforming the barriers to educational mobility will accommodate learning needs and career goals of our future students. The barriers are not in our educational institutions, not in our students, but in ourselves. Thus, so are the solutions. Solutions to transform barriers to educational mobility in nursing include:

1. Partnerships with nursing service to support mobility for employed nurses and assistants. A number of model projects exist; for example, New York's Project L.I.N.C. in which the Greater New York Hospital Association and City nursing schools offer special programs whereby nursing attendants, LPNs, RNs, and BSNs can advance educationally and within their nursing career. The University of San Francisco and a nearby Kaiser Foundation Hospital jointly support a class of Kaiser RN employees toward a BS degree through specially scheduled part-time study. Nursing homes in California support classes of nursing assistants enrolled part-time in practical nurse programs, and two groups of LPN employees enrolled in two ADN programs in specially scheduled part-time programs.
2. Continued work on differentiation of pre-licensure content in nursing is critical to overcoming the barriers. Agreement on content differences between programs diminishes the strength of traditional biases. Clarity and agreement in content differentiation also diminishes the need for pretesting as a part of enrolling students who have had previous nursing education, and increases the success of transition instruction by utilizing specially designed experiences which bridge segments.
3. Discretion, fairness, and flexibility need to be exercised in making decisions about upper- and lower-division courses and transfer credit. Many schools are successful in skillfully handling the system in order to facilitate articulation for qualified students.

4. We need activities which foster trust and clarity in order to achieve consistency and predictability. A successful example exists in the work of an ad hoc articulation committee in California, chaired by Marilyn Flood of University of California–San Francisco. It includes representatives from both BS and AD programs meeting periodically for more than a year, which has enlarged the level of understanding and trust among all the state's nurse educators.
5. Finally, we need to promote the view that nursing will survive—even flourish—with a pluralistic educational system. Academic integrity and the open curriculum are not mutually exclusive phenomena.

REFERENCES

Anderson, E. H. (1972, March). The associate degree program—A step to the baccalaureate degree? *Current Issues in Nursing Education.* New York: National League for Nursing. Papers presented at the Ninth Conference of the Council of Baccalaureate and Higher Degree Programs.

Boyle, R., Ren, E., & Paterson, F. K. (1962). The registered nurse seeks a college. *Nursing Outlook, 10,* 652–654.

Hansen, H. A. (1988, May). *A study of baccalaureate degree nursing program curricula in California.* ADN-BSN Articulation Committee of the California Association of Colleges of Nursing and the Associate Degree Nursing Directors of California.

Hodgkinson, H. L. (1985). *All one system: Demographics of education, kindergarten through graduate school.* Washington, DC: Institute for Educational Leadership.

Kibrick, A. (1968). Why collegiate programs for nurses? *New England Journal of Medicine, 278,* 765–772.

MacLean, T. B., Knoll, G. H., & Kinney, C. K. (1985). The evolution of a baccalaureate program for registered nurses. *Journal of Nursing Education, 2,* 53–57.

Matheney, R. V. (1975). Open curriculum—Yes! In C. B. Lenburg (Ed.), *Open learning and career mobility in nursing* (p. 85). St Louis: Mosby.

National League for Nursing. (1964). *Department of baccalaureate and higher degree programs statement of beliefs and recommendations regarding baccalaureate nursing programs admitting registered nurse students.* New York: National League for Nursing.

Reverby, S. (1987). *Ordered to care.* Cambridge University Press.

Sonoma State University. (1974). *Self study for accreditation by the National League for Nursing.* Rohnert Park, CA: Author.

Transforming the state role in undergraduate education. (1986, July 30). *The Chronicle of Higher Education,* pp. 14–15.

8

Alternatives for Students with Life Experiences: Reconceptualizing Nursing Education

Clair E. Martin, PhD, RN

The problem with our future is that it isn't what it used to be. Consequently, the customary methods of achieving our goals may not be productive. Visionary leadership which is capable of risk taking, must chart new courses for survival in a rapidly changing world. A strategy that projects an extension of the status quo, or simply reacts with a patchwork program, is not only unable to provide leadership, but will act to retard nursing's potential role in being part of the solution to the critical health care problems facing our nation. The cliche "If you're not part of the solution, you're part of the problem" may aptly be applied in light of the current crisis in health care.

Peters (1988) uses the phrase "Go to the sound of the guns" to challenge leaders to secure frontline information as the basis for proactive decision making. For nursing education, going to the sound of the guns means obtaining first-hand information from both our prospective students about their needs and potentials, and from nursing's patients and clients regarding their need for professional nursing care.

THE "NEW" NURSING STUDENTS

Who They Are and How We Can Help Each Other

The age and experience of prospective students is changing dramatically. The fastest growing cohort of the student population is age 35 or over ("Education department," 1988). Paradoxically, the traditional 18 to 22-year-old white female student may well be the unusual student of tomorrow. This change in student characteristics is the consequence of social forces that will profoundly influence the structure, content, and processes of our curricula. Many of our students have postsecondary credentials and degrees in nursing or other fields. (For the purpose of this chapter the student who has a postsecondary certificate or degree in either nursing or another area is described as the student with life experience.) This year 35 percent of the students entering their junior year in the Nell Hodgson Woodruff School of Nursing at Emory University already hold a degree in another field. The needs and potentials of these students are considerably different from the class of 10 years ago. Hodgkinson (1985) says that changes in the composition of today's student population "will change the system faster than anything else except nuclear war" (p. 1).

On the other hand, patients today require professional nurses to demonstrate a higher level of critical thinking and clinical judgment than ever before. The tomorrow envisioned by futurists will be even more complex, challenging professional nursing to higher levels of expertise and competence (Warnick, 1988).

The student with postsecondary credentials is a potential—or at least partial—solution to both the quantity and quality needs of professional nursing. To realize the potentials represented by these students, nursing education is challenged to design educational programs that are responsive to the unique needs of these students and maximize the potential of their learning experiences. Times of crisis are actually opportunities for change insofar as customary behaviors are often not productive in goal attainment under these conditions. The current supply/demand imbalance in nursing provides an atmosphere of receptivity to creatively designed programs that might not be present in times of relative stability. Although securing a supply/demand balance must include utilization studies that address safe, cost-effective alternatives which reduce nurse time spent in peripheral non-nursing activities, the focus of this chapter is on the supply-side potential of a largely untapped cohort of prospective nurses.[1]

Recruiting adequate numbers of qualified professional nurses is a major challenge facing nursing today. Previous recruitment strategies were directed toward high school graduates, for whom nursing education was simply an extension of their primary and secondary education. This strategy worked when the demographic profile looked like a pyramid, but

[1] Simply increasing the supply of nurses to reduce the immediate crisis will not resolve the cyclic pattern of shortages. Profound changes in the autonomy, rewards, and status afforded nurses must be attained. In this respect, an exclusive focus upon supply simply retards resolution of the problem and is a self-defeating strategy.

with an aging population, the largest population cohort is middle-aged. In addition, many students discovered previously unavailable career opportunities, and interest in nursing declined while the proportion of nontraditional students interested in nursing increased.

The profession has both the obligation and the privilege of selecting and socializing its new members. This social contract allows those in positions of power considerable autonomy to establish the admission, progression, and graduation requirements within the professional curricula as well as regulate the entry of new practitioners. This privilege is contingent upon the profession's commitment to prepare adequate numbers of competent practitioners to meet societal needs. The current shortage emphasizes the need to address both the quantity and quality of professional nurses.

Quantity

A closer look at the issue of quantity reveals that the Bureau of Labor projects an increase of 43.6 percent in new registered nurse positions by the year 2000 (Silvestri & Lukasiewicz, 1987). While the Division of Nursing projects a relative balance between supply and demand in the year 2000, this probably underestimates total demand and certainly does not reveal the undersupply for baccalaureate- and higher-degree-prepared nurses. The changes which occurred after 1982 in the health care delivery system have dramatically increased the demand for the higher-degree-prepared nurse. Therefore, a shortfall of baccalaureate- and higher-degree-prepared nurses is projected (Department of Health and Human Services, 1988).

A significant increase in the proportion of high school graduates enrolled in nursing is unlikely, given the opportunities for women in other careers and the resistance to making nursing more attractive for men. In addition, the high school population is increasingly nonwhite. Traditionally, blacks and Hispanics have not participated in higher education to the same extent as their white counterparts. Thus even if an increased proportion of high school graduates is enrolled, the population will not be able to provide an adequate supply. The number of high school graduates peaked at 3.2 million in 1977 and will drop to 2.4 million in 1992 (Department of Health and Human Services, 1988). The bulge in the population profile is in the 35–45-year-old cohort. Many members of this group will consider a second career, which, along with recruitment of traditional high school graduates, will hopefully work to meet the total quantity needs for professional nurses.

Multiple career changes have already become a pattern. Each year one-third of the American work force changes jobs, and it is predicted that most of this population will pursue four to five different careers during their lifetimes (Naisbitt & Aburdene, 1985). According to Jung's theoretical formulations of human development, individuals approaching midlife appraise their current situations in terms of total life goals. Most individuals find it both necessary and easier to pursue selected interests and develop those abilities that facilitate achievement of goals early in life. In other terms most individuals develop either a left-brain or right-brain modus operandi. At midlife there is a felt pressure to achieve a balance. One possible consequence of the midlife appraisal is to develop the "shadow side" (Jung, 1971). As applied to nursing, insofar as this theoretical formulation is valid, the internalized utilitarian cultural values of a "me" generation that influenced career decisions are subject to challenge at midlife. Provided an opportunity to perceive professional nursing as a way to articulate earlier life experiences in a meaningful way, individuals considering a second career may find in nursing and its humanistic "other" orientation the potential for developing their shadow side and achieving the desired balance.

The social fact of multiple career changes paralleled by the psychological needs of midlife represents an opportunity for nursing to expand its recruitment to meet the desired quantity and quality of practitioners. In addition, this cohort may also have a vested interest in assuring adequate care for the rapidly expanding aging population.

Quality

The desired qualities of the professional nurse represent the most intriguing rationale for designing nursing education programs in light of and in harmony with the needs and potentials represented by experienced students. The "Essentials" report (American Association of Colleges of Nursing, 1986) outlines a comprehensive set of expectations for the education of the professional nurse. Unquestionably the knowledge, abilities, professional behaviors, and values set forth are desirable and necessary assets for the beginning professional nurse. However, given the time limitations of an undergraduate degree, the opportunity to secure depth of understanding and commitment is limited. On the other hand, students building on a postsecondary credential have a greater potential for demonstrating the understanding and ability prescribed by this report.

Schlotfeldt's (1988) presentation to the 1988 Dean's Summer Seminar is both illustrative and challenging in its conception of the professional nurse role. She says:

> Scholarly nursing practitioners carry awesome responsibilities . . . [and] should be broadly educated in the several fields of human knowledge and be capable of developing interests and attitudes, as well as career aspirations that enable them to provide intimate helping services to fellow human beings who need knowledgeable, sensitive, humane, and ethical care that fulfills a particular social mission. (pp. 19–20)

A rigorous professional program of study will enable the new professional

> . . . to articulate and to demonstrate the goal, focus, domain, and beneficial outcomes of their professional services; they are competent and self-confident in promoting nursing care in any setting and in any field of differentiated general nursing practice . . . should demonstrate the ability to engage in systematic inquiry and the habits of the mind that lead them toward continuous learning and toward orchestrating a productive career in a learned profession that has a multitude of career opportunities and plenty of room at the top. (Schlotfeldt, 1988, p. 20)

Too frequently, nurses, patients, and families recognize that available services are, unfortunately, inadequate. Students with life experience are a potential cohort to meet the qualitative requirements of professional practice.

CHANGING THE CURRICULUM FOR THE CHANGING STUDENT

To realize the potential this prospective pool of nurses represents, we must change our notions about the "right" curriculum. The student who has already experienced the autonomy, status, and rewards of a career is unlikely to willingly accept the powerless, low status role ascribed to students in our schools of nursing.

Nursing education has been less than enthusiastic in designing programs for these students, with a few notable exceptions. A recent survey of National League for Nursing accredited master's programs revealed that 97 percent of the respondents believed their programs to be traditional, although 36 percent stated they had nontraditional options (Forni, 1987). Carolyne Davis, Chairperson of the Secretary's Commission on Nursing, responded to the question, "What is your view of the world in terms of an ideal system of nursing education?" as follows:

> An ideal system of nursing education, in my view, would be much more flexible in terms of opportunity for educational advancement. I hope that the nursing education community will soon become more receptive to establishing nontraditional options. ("Carolyne Davis Speaks," 1988, p. 357)

The demand for educational programs for students with life experience is also cited as one of the top ten trends affecting nursing by the editors of *Nursing and Health Care* ("Ten Trends," 1986). Futurists Naisbitt and Aburdene (1985) state that we are spending as many dollars educating adults outside of traditional higher education institutions as within them, and project that this trend will increase.

The demand for educational innovation responsive to nontraditional student needs and potentials is significant, and the potential benefit to professional nursing of responding to this demand is equally so. Is nursing to take a visionary or reactive course? Creating a future that happens *for* nursing rather than *to* nursing is possible with a visionary commitment.

The experienced student can be an asset to the academic enterprise. In addition to generally being more motivated as a result of having clearer life goals, these students show more interest and enthusiasm for learning. Vicarious learning opportunities are clearly documented as a critical factor in student socialization. Bok (1986) suggests that the life experiences of these students can be an asset to teachers as well as to other students. He says:

> Much of the value of the undergraduate experience comes from the chance to know other people of widely varying backgrounds and talents . . . the presence of accomplished, experienced adults would add a unique resource for a community in which even faculty members may have led quite specialized, circumscribed lives. (p. 123)

The actual experience of innovative programs designed for students with life experience supports the assertion that they can be a partial solution to the quantity and quality needs for professional nursing. Presently, two schools, Case Western and Rush, offer a Nursing Doctorate (ND). Yale, Pace, Massachusetts General, Rush, University of Tennessee–Knoxville, and Vanderbilt offer a master's degree in nursing for non-nurse college graduates, with a number of other schools planning to implement similar programs as well. In addition, a number of programs offer RN-MN options or accelerated programs that offer a second baccalaureate degree in nursing.

Diers (1987) surveyed ten programs designed for college graduates. There were two types: accelerated programs that offered a second baccalaureate, and combined programs that offered a master's or ND degree after completion of a program of study that skips the BSN. All but two of these programs are located in private universities; most are small and enrollment is cut off at a fixed upper limit. In 1986, approximately half of the applicants to these programs were admitted. In both types of programs nearly all of the students who have enrolled graduate. The percentage of male applicants has been greater than in traditional baccalaureate programs. This survey indicates that enrollments peaked in 1983 and have since declined in a pattern paralleling the enrollment decline in traditional undergraduate nursing programs. Although this may seem discouraging, the survey also concluded that those who apply to these programs have a strong, positive image of nursing.

An evaluation of the Case Western Doctor of Nursing (ND) program revealed that ND graduates were significantly older than BSN graduates, a larger percentage were men, and 51 percent were single. ND graduates scored significantly higher on the N-CLEX than did BSN graduates. On the four subscales of the Characteristics of the Graduate Instrument there was no significant difference between ND and BSN graduates and on the Six-Dimension Scale of Nursing Performance, supervisors failed to note any differences in quality of performance. Both groups reported comparable feelings of overall satisfaction in their present positions. The survey found that 76 percent of the ND graduates planned on continuing nursing education compared to 37 percent of the BSN graduates (Fitzpatrick, Boyle, & Anderson, 1986). Clearly these innovative vanguard programs have demonstrated that a high quality competent professional nurse can be prepared in nontraditional ways.

RECOMMENDATIONS

There are a number of recommendations that I believe will enhance the appeal of nursing for students with life experience and will at the same time facilitate the achievement of the ideals of the curriculum revolution as presented in the Fourth and Fifth National Educators Conferences.

Humanizing Nursing Education

In a fundamental sense, humanizing nursing education begins with the recognition that both students and faculty bring life experiences that greatly influence the success potential of the teaching–learning venture. In an ideal teaching–learning situation, all of those involved are engaged in a process of becoming as they interdependently pursue discovery and learning. Although increasing numbers of students with life experience are enrolled in nursing education programs, their general experience with the available alternatives has been disenchanting. The increased interest is a greater tribute to the students' perceptions of opportunities available in professional nursing practice than to the congruence between experienced learning opportunities and their needs and interests. Too frequently the personal experience of these students is marked by hostility and alienation rather than partnership in a learning venture. Students feel compelled to "psych out" the teacher, repeat bits of information, and demonstrate behaviors they assume are expected of them. They feel that their past experiences are viewed as undesirable and threatening to the faculty and that the safest course of action is to dissociate themselves from their past. The status differential between student and teacher is profound, and the "bad" student is one who does not recognize his or her proper role. The distasteful phrase "Nursing eats its young" can credibly be applied to the felt experiences of many of these students. The irony is that generally the faculty's felt experience is no more positive than the student's.

Why does this mutually alienating experience occur so frequently? Why isn't there greater congruence between student learning needs and the program structure, content, and processes they confront? I believe that at least one factor is our world view perspective about education. We assume that the Tyler model which emphasizes technically oriented goals and objectives is the proper education model. This model inhibits our ability to articulate new learning challenges for these students and emphasizes repetition.

Bevis described the Tyler model as based on behaviorist learning theory.

> Behavioral objectives as the sole arbiters of learning are too narrow and lack the creative energy necessary to guide the awakening discovery that must mark true education. Behavioral objectives represent minimal achievement levels, and are effective primarily for skill training and instruction. But they are not useful for seeing patterns and finding meanings, for enculturation into the profession or for learning the creative strategies necessary to identify, classify, and solve the problems of the discipline. They stifle creativity and provide restrictive guides for evaluations. (Bevis, 1988, pp. 33–34)

The opportunity to develop the critical thinking, clinical judgment, and values of social responsibility essential to a practice discipline is shortchanged in this model. Its rigid structure inhibits the integration of past experiences and restricts the potential to exploit the phenomenological learning opportunities arising from current interests and experiences. It is no wonder that these students feel disengaged and impotent to participate in their own education. Both faculty and students assume that it is inappropriate to pursue subjects that are not covered by a behavioral objective properly ordered on a course syllabus.

Diekelmann (1988) challenges nursing educators to address processes that empower students through dialogue, to provide greater opportunity to think critically, and to pursue learning as it is relevant to the students' needs and interests. These processes have the potential of reconciling the teacher and student in a relationship of mutual respect where both are interdependent learners. Nowhere in nursing education is there a greater need for such reconciliation than in relation to students who bring life experiences to their learning. Rather than being an asset, life experiences become a burden to both the teacher and the student if not dealt with in a positive way. These students, like all of us, must constantly unlearn as well as learn. However, it is difficult to conceive of a student who does not have prior experience that can be a supportive foundation for professional learning.

Harmful Language

Our ambiguous labeling of nursing programs can confuse both prospective students and the general public. Hart and Sharp's (1987) plea to abandon the terms generic, or first and second professional degree, in favor of a straightforward descriptive typology should be supported. The knowledge, skills, and attitudes expected of a person who holds an associate, baccalaureate, master's, or doctoral degree are considerably more significant than the trajectory of their student career. This change reflects a goal orientation that will reduce the confusion resulting from an emphasis upon the multiple pathways of *how* persons become prepared for a particular role rather than a focus upon *who* they have become. To the extent that our education system remains idiosyncratic to nursing, public understanding will be lacking and prospective students (especially those most likely to opt for nontraditional pathways) will be less likely to pursue a career in nursing. We must work to become goal oriented and put our programs within the context of mainstream education.

Accreditation

The purpose of accreditation is to assure the public that academic integrity and quality are maintained. However, the latent function of accreditation is the maintenance of the status quo. Emphasis upon "the right way" constrains experimentation or at least inhibits visibility of innovation as schools seek to protect their accreditation status. In this case, what people believe to be real, ie., the belief that there is a rigid set of interpretations of the accreditation criteria, is real in its consequences.

Diekelmann (1988) suggests that a process be designed that would enable schools to petition the National League for Nursing to suspend particular accreditation criteria and to substitute other criteria that would permit experimentation with models other than the Tyler model. What process would secure the quality goal of accreditation while encouraging the demonstration of alternatives? Risk taking and the willingness to be wrong do not come easily in nursing, but are essential in light of the rapidly changing context within which nursing education occurs. Now is the time to allow schools to demonstrate that academic integrity can be achieved and maintained in radically different ways.

Faculty Development

The success of the curriculum revolution is dependent upon an increase in self-esteem, the personal and collective empowerment that promotes appreciation of and commitment to risk taking. A positive sense of personal and collective esteem will also promote the teacher–student relationship as one of interdependent learners engaged in mutual discovery. Learning that is oriented to the interests and needs of the student and that reflects his or her cognitive style is also more likely in this environment. Experienced students will be a challenge to faculty.

Profiling stories of individuals or schools who have successfully implemented innovations will provide positive feedback and encouragement for those considering taking a risk. Faculty development programs that provide knowledge of alternative curricular models and humanistic teaching strategies can increase the congruence between the reality of the teaching–learning situation and the ideal envisioned by the faculty member. Reducing this discrepancy between the real and the ideal works to increase self-esteem.

Faculty place a high value on the teacher–student relationship. Their intent is to create learning situations that are positive experiences for the student. However, it is generally understood that faculty are most likely to teach what they have been taught in the way they have been taught. There is a collective perception that this is the way it should be. Faculty workshops and clinics that provide the opportunity to understand and demonstrate new behaviors congruent with the ideals of the curriculum revolution must be provided and recognition for successful innovation should be broadly publicized.

Recruitment

A significant increase in enrollment of students with life experiences in nursing schools has occurred without a marketing program aimed toward them. A plan which is nationally visible and designed to familiarize mature, second-career students with the opportunities available in nursing education and practice should be initiated.

Major employers should be familiarized with the opportunities nursing offers second-career students. Technological advances will increasingly reduce demand for certain categories of personnel. (For example, computers will soon do the majority of their own programming.) In this case, monitoring changing work force requirements could provide a focus for targeted recruiting. Also, economic realities often require people who reach retirement to continue working. The Armed Forces are a major employer and substantial numbers of people retire from active duty, many of whom have received a baccalaureate degree at taxpayers' expense. If the Armed Forces were committed to a program such as this, successful recruitment of substantial numbers of students with life experience who would meet a critical national need would hopefully occur. A major concern of the Armed Forces is securing an adequate supply of professional nurses for both active and reserve duty. Therefore, the Armed Forces could be both a major supplier of students with life experience to innovative nursing programs and a major beneficiary of these programs. In any case, new, creative approaches to recruiting the student with life experience must be designed and implemented.

Admissions

Unnecessary admission hurdles need to be reduced. One significant hurdle is the use of standardized tests. Standardized test scores predict little enough of the prospective student's academic performance and have less value in identifying what the student will contribute in his or her professional career (Bok, 1986). On the other hand, these tests are a significant source of anxiety for the experienced student and as such are a disincentive. Is the time, cost, and anxiety of these admission tests warranted in terms of their limited predictive value? It is time to re-evaluate the extent to which these tests are able to facilitate the selection of qualified students who will make a professional contribution. Demonstrated academic ability and clear professional goals are much more significant in determining potential professional contribution.

Financial Support

Broader sources of financial support are necessary. For the most part, students with life experience have ongoing family and/or economic responsibilities that require financial support for their education. The ratio of loans to scholarships must also be taken into account; having a significant debt at midlife would be a major disincentive. While increased federal programs are necessary, the primary source of financial support could be through agreements between the school offering the program and the service organizations which would employ the graduates.

Center for Innovation in Nursing Education

No matter how significant the Fourth and Fifth Conferences have been in increasing faculty and administration understanding of the ideals of the curriculum revolution, unless the ideals are kept visible, it is likely that the status quo will remain. The conference theme "Curriculum Revolution" suggests a dramatic departure from the usual and customary, requiring at the very least an objective analysis of current curricula and their implementation.

Van Oech (1983), in his creative monograph titled, *A Whack on the Side of the Head,* describes ten attitudes that interfere with the generation of innovation and that reinforce the status quo. The curriculum revolution is inhibited by the widespread belief that: (a) there is a right answer, (b) the rules must be followed, and (c) to err is wrong. The attendance at these conferences suggests that there is a strong desire for curriculum to be different in both structure and process. However, the inertia of the status quo can be overcome only through the continuing visibility, dialogue, and legitimization of alternatives.

Establishing a Center for Innovation in Nursing Education located within the NLN structure could be a valuable and necessary structural asset in promoting the ideals presented at the Fourth and Fifth Educators Conferences.

The first function of the center would be to visibly legitimate innovation and change and to challenge and support programs in the exploration and demonstration of options. It would facilitate recruitment by profiling successful students and graduates. Prospective students who may not otherwise consider a career in nursing may be motivated to do so as a result of their ability to identify with someone who has been successful.

The center's public relations effort would serve to sensitize the industry to opportunities within nursing education to re-educate workers whose positions are being phased out or who are retiring. In our rapidly changing economy these situations will occur with increasing frequency. It would also sponsor think tanks to identify strategies for integrating the life experiences of students and for maximizing their professional knowledge and skill. Multi-institutional grant proposals to demonstrate the effectiveness of innovations could be orchestrated along with a plan to broadly disseminate the project findings.

Another primary function would be to coordinate faculty development efforts in keeping with the structural and process innovations in curriculum. A network of consultants and workshop leaders would support faculty development.

The basic structure of this center differs significantly from Mitchell's (1988) proposal for a Center for Alternative Nursing Education in several ways. What I propose is a broadly decentralized movement that is supported from the legitimate base of the NLN. (The word alternative connotes a secondary type effort.) What I propose is a structured vehicle to facilitate the curriculum revolution to the extent that its humanizing ideals become the mainstream.

SUMMARY

A future that happens *for* nursing will be created only if visionary nurses provide the necessary leadership. The experienced student is potentially part of the solution to our need for professional nurses, in terms of both quantity and quality. There is an obvious connection between recognizing the needs and potentials of students with life experience and the ideals of the curriculum revolution. In fact, it is possible that the student with life experience could be considered one of the motivating forces that drives the curriculum revolution toward its eventual victory.

REFERENCES

American Association of Colleges of Nursing. (1986). *Essentials of college and university education for professional nursing.* Washington, DC: American Association of Colleges of Nursing.

Bevis, E. O. (1988). New directions for a new age. In *Curriculum revolution: Mandate for change* (pp. 27–52). New York: National League for Nursing.

Bok, D. (1986). *Higher learning.* Cambridge, MA: Harvard University Press.

Carolyne Davis speaks out. (1988, September). *Nursing and Health Care, 9*(7), 355–359.

Department of Health and Human Services. (1988). *Secretary's Commission on Nursing Interim Report.* Washington, DC: U.S. Government Printing Office.

Diekelmann, N. (1988). Curriculum revolution: A theoretical and philosophical mandate for change. In *Curriculum revolution: Mandate for change* (pp. 137–158). New York: National League for Nursing.

Diers, D. (1987). When college grads choose nursing. *American Journal of Nursing, 87*(12), 1631–1637.

Education department foresees slight fluctuations in number of college students over next decade. (1988, November). *Chronicle of Higher Education,* pp. 1, A33–34.

Fitzpatrick, J. J., Boyle, K. K., & Anderson, R. M. (1986). Evaluation of Doctor of Nursing (ND) program: Preliminary findings. *Journal of Professional Nursing, 2*(6), 365–372.

Forni, P. R. (1987). Nursing's diverse master's programs: The state of the art. *Nursing and Health Care, 8*(2), 71–75.

Hart, S., & Sharp, T. G. (1987). Harmful to our health: The language of nursing education. *Nursing and Health Care, 8*(4), 229–231.

Hodgkinson, H. L. (1985). *All one system: Demographics of education—kindergarten through graduate school.* Washington, DC: Institute for Educational Leadership.

Jung, C. G. (1971). *The portable Jung* (J. Campbell, Ed.; R. F. C. Hull, Trans.). New York: Penguin.

Mitchell, C. A. (1988). One view of the future: Nontraditional education as the norm. *Nursing and Health Care, 9*(4), 187–190.

Naisbitt, J., & Aburdene, P. (1985). *Re-inventing the corporation.* New York: Warner.

Peters, T. (1988). *Thriving on chaos.* New York: Alfred A. Knopf.

Schlotfeldt, R. M. (1988). The scholarly nursing practitioner. In C. A. Lindeman (Ed.), *Alternate conceptions of work and society: Implications for professional nursing.* Washington, DC: American Association of Colleges of Nursing.

Silvestri, G. T., & Lukasiewicz, J. M. (1987). A look at occupational employment trends to the year 2000. *Monthly Labor Review,* 46–63.

Ten trends to watch. (1986, January). *Nursing and Health Care, 7*(1), 16–19.

von Oech, R. (1983). *A whack on the side of the head.* New York: Warner.

Warnick, M. (1988). The delphi survey. In D. Smith (Ed.), *Nursing 2020: A study of the future of hospital-based nursing* (pp. 49–50). New York: National League for Nursing.

9

The Curriculum Consequences: Aftermath of Revolution

Em Olivia Bevis, MA, RN, FAAN

REVOLUTIONS ARE FEARSOME BEASTS

Revolutions scare me. They are often bloody and destructive, accompanied by the sound of bombs and followed by the hush of silence after destruction. They are a time of noise, waste, and devastation . . . a time when passion rules and reason abdicates. They are fearsome beasts resembling the flesh-eating Tasmanian devils. All too often, the world is not a better place when the revolution is over; tyranny simply exists under another name. Consider world history and let the French la Guillotine, Oliver Cromwell, Lenin, Stalin, Mao, Franco, and Castro be witness for my claims.

Most revolutions have a few proletarian intellectuals who think they can control things. But revolutions are war, and in war only Ares and Eris, the gods of war and discord, rule. As a part of revolution, people of reason and wisdom are often martyred. After revolution there are periods of rigidly prescribed behaviors, and those who do not conform are discounted—and too often discontinued.

Given the social psychology of revolution, I prefer a longer period of planned change—not evolution, for that takes too long—but planned change. In this, we would set up tasks to be accomplished and establish task forces to work on them. Perhaps as we move toward new paradigms for curriculum development we will see an alteration in climate that will permit planned change rather than the chaos of revolution. However, for the purposes of this chapter, I must assume that we are dealing with a revolution, and I will attempt to help structure it to have as many of the positive and as few of the negative potential consequences of revolution as possible.

CONSTRUCTION: THE SUBLIME MISSION OF REVOLUTION

Divisiveness or Unity

As in any revolution, the revolt is not enough; the sublime mission is to construct. In order that it not be a null revolution, we must be very clear about how we know when the revolution is succeeding. Can revolutionaries disagree on the aftermath and still be successful? Or must all revolutions result in power struggles? Nursing's history is rife with class conflict. As an oppressed group with all the problems of oppression, we are always more ready to fight each other than to unite against a common threat.

We must break the barriers of social class stratification that divide us. The social status prejudices that exist among teachers of nursing spring from the same kind of ignorance and bigotry that support sexism, racism, and anti-Semitism. It is immoral and antithetical to our goals and we must not allow it to continue to flourish in our new world. We must value the strengths and contributions of each program so that all faculties—associate degree, diploma, baccalaureate, masters, and doctorate—participate together in shaping the revolution. Only in this way can we prevent the oppression inherent in class status from casting its dark shadow over the future. This evil carries in it the seeds of failure.

I am hopeful that developmentally we are outgrowing the factionalism that has plagued us and we can work together to plan an acceptable future. To do this we need some general agreement regarding what points of reference we can trust to tell us that we have not traded one tyranny for another but have actually succeeded in changing nursing education in ways that make us more able to meet the nursing needs of society in the 21st century. Notice that I said some general agreements. We do not want—nor do we need—rigid parameters that dictate content or process or prescribe curriculum elements.

Indicators of Success

What are we moving toward? What are we constructing? What characteristics will distinguish the new from the old? These are questions that must be answered now—not at the end—for these answers become both the goals of the revolution and the criteria of success.

Assumptions about the Future

Before launching my projections about the new world of nursing education it is necessary to comment about some of the assumptions regarding the future world in which nursing will exist:

1. The three major sources of health problems of the next 30 years are likely to be the great increases in the population of the eldest el-

derly, prolonged survival of more health-threatened people which will radically increase the numbers of the chronically ill, and the growing number of people with AIDS. All three of these are problems for which nursing care is *the* major health industry provider. Therefore it can be assumed that the need for nursing care will rise logarithmically, and nursing personnel shortages will continue to be an industry problem.

2. Medical science has brought us to impossible choices that disturb our deepest sense of ethics and our moral commitments as nurses. Our ability to enable more people to live out the full extent of human life expectancy has had a major effect on the strains now placed upon society's and nursing's ability to cope with the numbers of persons needing health and nursing care. As a result we can make the following assumptions:

   A. Practicing nurses must be ethically grounded and be perspicacious, wise, and compassionate in order to shoulder their share of responsibility for the morality of health care.

   B. Medical science will continue to place emphasis upon high levels of technology. Nurses must not only be able to work effectively in these technically complex environments, but be able to humanize these environments with caring and concern so that clients are persons not objects of health care.

   C. The strains of aging, chronicity, and AIDS will so stress the health care system and the country's precarious fiscal balance that survival of capitalistic democracy will require a total shift in the health care paradigm. Nursing will need to assume a major role in the restructuring process both in policy setting and in care delivery.

Implications of Assumptions

As a consequence of these factors, nursing education is required to provide society with nurses who are highly educated, highly skilled scholar-clinicians in sufficient numbers to rise to the task of fulfilling the roles ascribed by the social mandate. Any revolution that fails to be attentive to these needs will render nursing impotent to deal with the needs of society and individuals, and nurses will be a footnote to history rather than one of the main players. Therefore, the revolution must result in substantive changes—changes that alter the nature of the graduate and provide the graduate with the skills, tools, and creative thinking necessary to be autonomous, imaginative, inventive, flexible, caring, ethical professionals committed to the whole range of possibilities from national policy setting to patient care.

Graduate characteristics are a result of two things: the type of student that is recruited and the curriculum of the student's education. I shall address curriculum first because studies show that students change as a result of schooling. Note the work done on the influence of formal higher education on moral reasoning. Felton and Parsons (1984) found that education had a significant impact on overall ethical/moral reasoning levels. This supported previous research findings reported by Rest (1979) that education is a significant variable in the development of ethical/moral reasoning. Additionally, the research revealed that neither socioeconomic level nor years of work experience were significantly related to ethical and moral reasoning. Furthermore, the findings indicated that stabilization of ethical/moral development occurs at the point one leaves formal education and that the educational experience may counteract moral and ethical reasoning that is influenced by work experience. One might surmise that ethical and moral reasoning would be the most difficult aspect of adults to alter, but these two studies indicate that this is not true and that education has a significant impact.

If it is true of ethical and moral reasoning, it follows that it is probably true of other important characteristics. Certainly the Edwards Personal Preference Inventory I used in two very different baccalaureate programs to determine changes in student characteristics during their nursing education showed definitive shifts in several areas.

Therefore, I shall first take as indicators of success, curriculum factors that find some agreement among those of my colleagues who are outspoken in their support of the curriculum revolution. Then I will look to other areas.

CRITERIA BASED ON APPARENT AGREEMENT

I think it important to note here that educators working on new paradigms for curriculum development in nursing are in agreement about some general directions. Some of these may be the material from which indicators of success are drawn.

One of these common agreements is basic to the whole paradigm shift that this revolution is about. It is something I hold as first principle (not as criteria): that any and all changes in paradigm must in some way affect the liberation and empowerment of people—both students and teachers. It is an indisputable theme in our revolution literature, in our discussion groups, and in our examples.

I raise the question: Is power of limited quantity so that when I empower others (students) I disempower myself? Or is power, like love, of unlimited quantity, so that the more I share the more I have. And through empowering others I also empower myself. I am attempting to think, not about "power over" but "power to." If power is conceived as "power to," then students and teachers are both empowered by the liberating force of co-learnership.

Curriculum as Teacher–Student Interactions or Dialogue

The most common agreement seems to be that curriculum is what actually occurs between and among persons in the educational enterprise and not some "plan" for learning that is reflected in written materials. Diekelmann (1988) states in her Dialogue and Meaning model that "curriculum is a dialogue among teachers, practitioners, and students on what will constitute the knowledge in the nursing curriculum and what role experience will play in the curriculum" (p. 144). She goes on to say that "dialogue is a joint reflection on a phenomenon; it is a deepening of experience for all participants; it is talking, generating questions, and possibly interpreting" (p. 145). Moccia (1988) asserts that "it is time for us to turn back to the swamp of interpersonal relations between student and teacher. It is time to focus on the process of education—the student–teacher relationship—rather than on its content or anything else" (p. 59). In this same article she states: "It is the authentic dialogue between people that makes any activity worthwhile, regardless of whether or not it is called successful by others" (p. 60).

Watson (1988) in addressing the University of Colorado proposed nurse doctorate program, stated that the change must "acknowledge faculty development needs for new teaching–learning methods and student–teacher interactive practices—e.g., shift from oppressive interactions to liberating interactions (or from maintenance learning to anticipatory-participatory learning) or emphasize faculty's role as expert learners rather than expert givers of information" (p. 4). Munhall (1988), in what she labels "Implications for Curriculum Within the Theme of the Aquarian Conspiracy," lists fostering community and searching for meaning, self-discovery, freedom, choices, and relationships as suggested processes. The implication here is that these processes are essential to the curriculum revolution. Bevis (1988) goes so far as to define curriculum as those transactions and interactions that take place between and among students and teachers with the intent that learning take place. She refers to Huebner's (1966) "opportunities for engagement" and believes that such opportunities are the material from which curriculum is made. She also states that "any mode of conceptualizing the nursing teacher's role in an authoritarian, frontal teaching, information-giving, control-laden way (ultimately politically oppressive) is antithetical to the caring paradigm that is nursing's moral imperative and nursing education's moral activity (which must be ultimately politically liberating)" (p. 22).

It seems, therefore, that a very high priority criterion is that the essence of curriculum rests in the quality of interactions between and among students and faculty. Professional educational programs rely on a changed relationship between teachers and students where the teacher's role is one of meta-strategist who raises questions and issues and dialogues with students so that they become partners in education not objects of education.

Curriculum That Stresses Syntactical Learning

A second criterion revolves around what students think about. The present paradigm for education is content laden—so content laden, in fact, that students have little time to think. Bevis (1988) writes:

> The mind is an awesomely powerful instrument. It can evoke memories that are as real and alive and full of feeling as the day of their occurrence. It can enact plans that are years in the making and complex in their execution. It can yearn, dream, imagine, envision, expunge, and intuit. It can follow a trail of clues so thin that there is hardly a smell of reality and leap through a chain of logic confounding in its convolutions. Its only limits are our inadequacy in its use, our unskilled handling of its superb potential, our waste of its vast abilities, our lack of vision of its limitless powers.
>
> In classes, we teachers reduce it to its most elementary functions: absorption, memorization, and recitation. We give lectures on the mistaken assumption that if the students don't hear us say it they will not learn it. We assume further that lecture is the most effective and efficient way to teach. Lecture is oppressive and in most cases inadequate. (p. 20)

(Though I will go on record as believing lecture is a good tool for a limited number of things, it would be tangential to elaborate here.)

Therefore, a second criterion for our revolution's success would be that faculty use teaching methodologies that stress syntactical learning which is characterized by viewing wholes, having insights and finding meanings, evaluating and projecting, and predicting from knowns to unknowns using both data and intuition. This type of learning enables people to make intuitive leaps and to trust them. It involves welding together theory and practice into praxis and helping students find practice-grounded patterns, examples, and models that support formation of personal general guides and paradigms and provide help in knowing when and under what circumstances one departs from these.

Curriculum as Critical and Creative Thinking

Most authors of the curriculum revolution have syntactical learning, as described above, as a major focus of education for nurses. This primarily involves critical and creative thinking, the search for meanings. Diekelmann (1988), in speaking of strategies that can be used in the new curricula, addresses the link between language and thinking and believes that "helping students understand the critical processes clinicians and teachers bring to nursing will help them understand the nature of critical thinking in nursing practice" (p. 151). Obviously, the critical thinking I am referring to is not as it is usually perceived—e.g., orderly, logical, objective, and scientific—but as grounded in subjective experience that, as Carolyn Oiler Boyd says, "scorn definition, procedure, determination, and abstractions" (1988, p. 66).

The criterion that arises from this rumination is regarding what students think about. The content-backed curriculum must be deflated—slimmed down—unpacked. Content has continually been added to the curriculum but seldom deleted. Students are graduated tired, overworked, burned out, and undereducated. As aftermath of the revolution, there must be an emphasis on content as the vehicle for learning, not the driver and dictator of timing, methodology, interactions, and evaluation. In other words, the new paradigms, rather than content burdened, will be interactive and educational process centered and oriented toward creative and critical thinking.

Reality Based Learning: Being-in-the-World

Currently, curriculum is faith teaching. Teachers focus on content emanating from a string of questionable logic that dictates it be derived from philosophy, conceptual frameworks, program, level, and course objectives. The selected content, which is usually what faculty thinks is discipline sanctioned, is taught on the faith that students will need that chosen bit of information at some time in their careers.

This must change. To be successful, the curriculum revolution must be both effective in enabling faculties to derive content differently and successful in grounding the student learning experiences in reality. Boyd (1988), in speaking about phenomenology as a foundation for curriculum says: "Lived experience is the focus of attention in phenomenology. Experience is not what we think, but what we live through. It is existing in a world; and, in the phenomenological sense, communicates the indivisible experiencing subject and experienced object" (p. 69). Diekelmann approaches content or knowledge as both theoretical and practical. Regarding experience in nursing education, she maintains that it is "restructured from one of a place in which theory is matched or applied in a laboratory or clinical setting to one of being-in-the-world with patients and nurses through language" (1987, p. 3).

Tanner (1988) concludes her article "Curriculum Revolution: The Practice Mandate" by commenting: "I do not think of developing more elegant and detailed formal models to be passed on to the next generation of nurses, for them to take and apply in their practice. Rather, I am struggling with ways in which the concerns of practice can truly be addressed by our educational activities, where classroom learning might be the application of practice rather than the other way around" (p. 214). Benner (1984) believes that expert clinical teachers can best teach through presenting paradigm cases. She says that these paradigm cases transmit more than can be conveyed through abstract principles or guidelines. She states, "in order for students to learn from another person's paradigm case, they must actively rehearse or imagine the situation. Simulations can be even more effective because they require action and decisions from the learner" (p. 9).

What emerges in most of my colleagues' writings is a concern for relevance, reality, and practice, so that not only does theory inform practice but practice informs theory. There also emerges a commitment to content in nursing having a clinical base—a contextual reality. Students in such a model are not whisked around from clinical experience to clinical experience and bent and molded in an effort to correlate some ideal of "theory" to some ideal of "practice." Instead, theory and practice coalesce or merge in ways that are meaningful for grounding content so that the contextual rules have an opportunity to be tested in reality and surface as grist for dialogue and teacher–student and student–student interactions, thereby finding their acontextual component in developing experience/expertise.

Practicum Experiences

One tradition-defying statement by Benner (1984, p. 185) goes upstream against institutionalized policy. Approval and accrediting bodies positively forbid specialization at undergraduate levels. This injunction seems to have no basis in research. Benner suggests, based upon her research, that "early clinical specialization in one area might be extremely advantageous in that it would give students an opportunity to learn about the process of acquiring advanced clinical knowledge." What Benner may be counseling here has more to do with remaining in one clinical setting long enough to acquire a repository of paradigm experiences in order to learn the processes where by one develops expertise, than with undergraduate specialization as such. I believe that not only are we mistaken about the need for students to experience all major nursing specialty settings but it is detrimental to developing the clinical scholars we all desire.

Diekelmann (1988, p. 147) opposes the popular conception that classroom and clinical practice should be closely correlated. She states: "The objective of developing clinical expertise in students does not depend on a corresponding relationship between classroom and clinical instruction." Further to confound the traditionalist, Diekelmann continues: "Students need not have at least one experience in each specialty area, nor are particular specialty areas or experiences mandatory" (p. 148). She believes, as I do, that these choices are for students to make in collaboration with teachers and clinical specialists. If we do not treat students as co-equals in the educational process and dialogue with them about their options and the wisdom of their choices, how can we ever hope to graduate autonomous nurses? Our fifth criterion, then, would be that in the new era, clinical experiences will be chosen by students after dialogue with teachers, fellow students, and clinicians; according to where they may best obtain the experiences they need in order to learn what they need to learn.

The sixth also addresses the idea that flexibility, not rigidity, must be the rule. Individuality of student choices and needs will be in evidence so that not all students will be required to have the same or nearly the same learning experiences. Students might, if they like, pursue some clinical interest that will enable them to learn how to develop expertise.

Phenomenological Teaching Approaches

In new models, clinical practice realities become the modality for study and the approach is qualitative in methodology rather than quantitative. Phenomenology, hermeneutical analysis, poetics, and other qualitative methods form the teaching–learning modalities. Both Munhall (1988) and Watson (1985) speak of the phenomenological thrust of the "new" nursing. Watson, in speaking of the transpersonal caring relationship of the nurse, states:

> Human care can begin when the nurse enters into the life space or phenomenal field of another person, is able to detect the other person's condition of being (spirit, soul), feels this condition within him- or herself, and responds to the condition in such a way that the recipient has a release of subjective feelings and thoughts he or she had been longing to release. As such, there is an intersubjective flow between the nurse and patient (p. 63).

Munhall states that "the social humandate for change calls us to conspire together in the transformation of behavioristic, externally driven curriculum to one that focuses on expanding consciousness and the subjective and intersubjective experiences of being human" (p. 228).

Boyd in her paper "Phenomenology of Nursing" says:

> We stand vulnerably in the wake of a spiraling system of controls on human irregularity made possible by 'scientific progress.' For some of us, the human condition—what it means to exist, to be alive in a world seized by technology—is an appropriate, even important focus for nursing. Existentialism and phenomenology provide a lens. (1988, p. 66)

There is little doubt for me that both existentialism and phenomenology are the lenses through which our curricula will reach the goals of excellence in professional service. In essence, they give us intentionality, and they ground the curriculum in "being-in-the-world." Additionally, unlike the scientific, they give us flexibility—the justification for looking at unconcealing . . . at coming to know . . . at exploring together. These ideas are antithetical to the common scientific positions of right and wrong answers, categorization of humans, human predictability, and division into parts. These two modes, existentialism and phenomenology, express wholes and explore consciousness. In speaking of phenomenological themes and concepts, Boyd states,

> These themes provide an open framework descriptive of the nature of being human: the first distinguishing feature of the phenomenological perspective. Rather than starting with a philosophy and constructing a curriculum, phenomenology grounds us only in an understanding of the nature of being human. There are fewer linear, derived guidelines and prescriptives, more openness, and more constancy in processes of choice. (p. 67)

Benner, another of the leaders in the phenomenological movement in nursing, offers guidance for phenomenological teaching approaches. If one defines curriculum as teacher–student interactions, these methods become the essence of the revolution. Benner (1984, p. 9) makes the case that "the proficient clinician compares past whole situations with current whole situations." Wholeness is something the behaviorist–empiricist paradigms seldom examine. Further, she believes that paradigm cases can be used as case studies and can be taken up as paradigms by learners. She states, "simulations [using paradigm cases] provide the learner with opportunities to gain paradigm cases in a guided way."

Another phenomenological methodology, poetics, can be useful in teaching. Poetics is a natural outcome of phenomenology. Watson (1985, p. 92) addresses this when she characterizes poetizing as the "true vocation of the experiential phenomenologist." She builds her position on Levin (1983) and maintains that poetizing is "necessary in that transcendental depth phenomenology, if focused and reflective of depth human experiences, cannot be other than poetic." If our teaching is centered on helping students find meaning, then poetics is a necessary element. Watson goes on to say, "Poetic expression has the power to touch and move us, to open and transport us. Thus, the poetic quality is related to the experiential meaning and, indeed, deepens the meaning, the felt senses, so that there is increased openness to describe and preserve the truth and depth of the experience."

Phenomenology is grounded in reality, in wholes, in reflection, in insight, in everyday events. Such, too, is hermeneutics. Hermeneutic inquiry examines the textual or language-semantic structure of everyday practical activity. It begins in the everyday practical roles and functions of nursing—what nurses actually do. Using hermeneutics, teachers and students seek meaning through language about practice. Diekelmann, Benner, Allen, and Tanner are among those whose writings support hermeneutics as a nursing educational mode.

Therefore, the seventh criterion reads: Clinical and classroom learning methodologies are qualitative rather than quantitative. Phenomenology, hermeneutical analysis, poetics, and other qualitative methods based upon humanistic-existentialism form the teaching–learning modalities.

Caring as the Moral Imperative of Nursing Education

Another striking common element among the leaders of this revolution is the emphasis on caring. Fifteen years ago caring was a *persona non grata* in nursing. It implied sentimentality and a gushy, valentine approach to nursing. A few mavericks—Leinneger, Murray, Bevis, Watson, Ray, Glittengerg, Gardner, Gaut, Parse, Boyle, and Uhl—were puttering along, outside the mainstream, researching, writing, and speaking about caring. These pioneers all believed that caring was the central core of nursing and formed its moral structure. Since that time, research and writing about caring fill volumes and have revealed much about the nature of caring and its role in nursing and nursing education. Commitment to the centrality of caring to the curriculum revolution is evident in the work of Watson, Benner, Diekelmann, Bevis, and Munhall. Actually, if a vote were taken, I think most nurses would agree that caring holds and must continue to hold a dominant role in our philosophy, our research, and our practice. Therefore, it must pervade our curriculum.

Watson (1985) has put it very powerfully: "Caring is the moral ideal of nursing" (p. 29). That must be our driver, our monitor, our guide in curriculum matters. She goes on to say that the ends of caring are protection, enhancement, and preservation of human dignity. Her belief is capsulized in her statement that: "Nursing as a human science and human care is always threatened and fragile. Because human care and caring requires a personal, social, moral, and spiritual engagement of the nurse and a commitment to oneself and other humans, nursing offers the promise of human preservation in society." This is not hyperbole. In a world which is increasingly computer driven; machine run; and controlled, mechanistic, and scientific; a world where even our elementary and high schools are "competency" based (i.e., behavioristic), nursing may well be the sanctuary of those most capable of preserving, sustaining, and protecting our collective and individual humanity. Munhall (1988, p. 227) in effect supports this position when she says that "the language of caring, which has been confined to the private domain and largely to women, emerges now as an ethical principle grounded in the concept of social responsibility and the credo of nonviolence."

Caring is powerful. Benner (1984, p. 208) identified six qualities of power associated with the caring provided by nurses. These are transformative, integrative, advocacy, healing, participative/affirmative, and problem solving. Bevis (1982) says, "The process of caring is as central to nursing as problem solving or communicating. It is implied every time 'nursing care' is referred to. Instead of *nursing* care the emphasis in on nurse *caring*" (p. 127). Bevis identified caring as essential content in nursing curricula. She included the research by Murray and Bevis done in the 1970s on the nature of the caring process in a chapter in her curriculum book. Bevis (1988) pointed out that one of the primary responsibilities of teachers in the new curriculum is to nurture the caring role. Diekelmann agrees, stating that, "The focus of the curriculum is the struggle to understand nursing knowledge and nursing practice. Caring, as an ontologic state, is fundamental to the curriculum" (1988, p. 144).

Therefore the eighth criterion is caring, as the moral ideal of nursing pervades the curriculum and forms its ethical imperative. It is the philosophical, research, and practice embodiment of nursing's essence and the source of nursing power. It is reflected in nursing's response to society's needs and its commitment to humanitarian service. Without caring, nursing is not a humanistic professional service, but a series of mechanistic tasks.

CRITERIA BASED ON COMMON SENSE

There are several criteria that arise not so much from agreement among leadership as from common sense. Some of these have received attention from voices of the revolution, some have received none. However, the mainstream of higher education, the history of nursing as a unified discipline, and the direction of flow of the discipline's growth each provide some evidence regarding indicators of success.

Professional Education is Based in the Arts and Humanities

In our search for legitimacy with our academic colleagues, nursing's movement from hospitals to academic settings was accompanied by a strong reliance upon empiricism and behaviorism. Nursing needed to be in control of its own practice, education, and research, and this required movement into settings of higher education. Additionally, nurse educators thought that to be acceptable in these settings, they had to assume the shape and texture of scientific academicians. So our art, so treasured in hospital curricula, gave way to science, so treasured in college curricula.

As we have become more self-confident, we have relinquished our drive to be an "applied" science and developed our own unique science—a human science. It is based upon an entirely different set of assumptions that match our mission and are holistic, humanistic, feminist, service-related, and ethical. These assumptions arise from a caring ethic, a humanities base, and an intersubjective reality of being in-the-world. This is at the very heart of the paradigm shift that motivates our revolution.

Sakalys and Watson (1985) reviewed seven major studies of education done in the 1980s. From these reports, they drew commonalities in curricular recommendations. First among these was "restoration of the centrality of the liberal arts in elementary, secondary, post-secondary, and professional education." In other words, there was an overriding concern for liberal arts within all the major studies and reports done on higher education in the first half of the 1980s.

Watson (1988) cites as one of the essentials for this transition the fact that we "acknowledge the arts and humanities as essential for educated persons and caring professionals." Her proposal for the nurse doctorate at the University of Colorado has a "more extensive liberal arts foundation" as its first principle. One of Boyd's concluding recommendations in her "Phenomenology for Nursing" (1988) is, not surprisingly, to "expand the use of the humanities in the nursing process."

I believe we have stressed the sciences at the expense of humanities too long in nursing. The tradition of Florence Nightingale is one of the liberally educated woman. Following this model, nurses would be classically educated prior to entering nursing. Today, instead of a classical education, we usually require two to four courses in chemistry, two in anatomy and physiology, two in psychology (usually general introduction and pathology), two in math (general algebra and statistics), and one each in growth and development, sociology, nutrition, microbiology, and occasionally physics. Students are usually allowed to choose *one* humanities course among speech, art appreciation, music appreciation, and philosophy. They are required to take some literature, and this nod toward the great thoughts of human history is considered enough—not only for nursing students but for most undergraduates in colleges and universities today.

Art, literature, poetry, music, philosophy, and architecture impart wisdom. They speak to that universal experience of humankind that unites and harmonizes. In the metaphors of art, poetry, music and architecture, human suffering and transcending courage find their expression. Compassion and identification with the progress of human thought comes through literature and philosophy. Science may give us the tools for curing, but it is the humanities that give us the tools for caring. When we put a humanities base in nursing curriculum, we elevate nursing to its place in human concerns and empower it, as Watson (1985) says, truly to protect, enhance, and preserve human dignity. More than that, we as nurses can be persuasive in preserving humanness in the healing technological jungle.

Therefore, the ninth criterion is that the curriculum include courses in art, music, literature, and philosophy. Additionally, nursing content should be approached using a humanities perspective.

Accessibility and Flexibility

The nudge toward accessibility and flexibility comes from the nature of the present world of students. Based on first-time candidates or the

July 1988 NCLEX, associate degree programs now graduate 57 percent and diploma programs 10 percent of the total. This means that about 67 percent of new nurses lack the first professional degree. Increasing numbers of students no longer enter the profession immediately after high school; many are reentry persons with either second careers or second degrees, and more students than ever before work 20 or more hours per week. These realities force nurse educators to plan programs that allow ADN graduates to seek baccalaureate degrees with the least possible problems, roadblocks, and redundancy. It forces us to examine and to reconstruct our programs of study in such areas as the policies governing entry, part-time study, scheduling, articulation, and challenge exams or transfer of credit. We must arrange our programs so that they are flexible and accessible. Further, our courses and treatment of students must acknowledge that a large number of our students are adults with whom we should interact as adult to adult and in ways that enrich both the student and the teacher.

The tenth criterion is that policies, guidelines, and programs of study are formulated in ways that provide for flexibility and accessibility in order to respond to the needs of the associate degree and other nontraditional students. The eleventh is that course construction and teacher–student interactions are forged in ways that acknowledge the adult nature of the learner.

NONCURRICULUM INDICATORS OF SUCCESS

Curriculum is not the only thing that must change in order for the new era to arrive. Other conditions are necessary to success. Three that can be viewed with a sense of certainty that the curriculum revolution is accomplishing its goals are paradigm-free accreditation and approval criteria and procedures, faculty development and education in new age teaching modalities, and alteration in the health care practice environments.

Paradigm-Free Accreditation and Approval Criteria

It is almost embarrassing to say the obvious, but to omit it would be presumptuous. All these ideals of the revolution are of no use unless we are unable to alter the criteria for national accreditation and state approval so that we can have indicators of excellence rather than paradigm-related criteria. Almost all state boards of nursing have—not in their nurse practice acts but in their rules and regulations governing educational programs—criteria that require that the products of the Tylerian/behavioristic/technological model be explicit in the curriculum-planning documents.

The National League for Nursing criteria for accrediting programs are also paradigm related. Though these criteria have, in the last two

FIRST PRINCIPLE

Any and all changes in paradigm must in some way affect the liberation and empowerment of people—both students and teachers.

CRITERIA

1. Professional educational programs rely on a changed relationship between teachers and students, wherein the teacher's role is one of meta-strategist who raises questions and issues and dialogues with students so that they become partners in education, not objects of education.
2. Faculty use teaching methodologies that stress syntactical learning which is characterized by viewing wholes, having insights, seeing patterns, finding meanings, evaluating, and predicting using both data and intuition.
3. Curriculum is interaction and educational process centered, and oriented toward creative and critical thinking not content burdened.
4. Clinical practice realities are the foci of study so that content in nursing has a contextual reality.
5. Clinical experiences are chosen by students after dialogue with teachers, fellow students, and clinicians, according to where they may best obtain the experiences they need.
6. Students need not all have similar learning experiences. Students may pursue some clinical interest that will enable them to learn how to develop expertise.
7. Phenomenology, hermeneutical analysis, poetics, and other qualitative methods based upon humanistic existentialism form the teaching–learning modalities.
8. Caring, as the moral ideal of nursing, pervades the curriculum and forms its ethical imperative. It is the philosophical, research, and practice embodiment of nursing's essence and the source of nursing power. It is reflected in nursing's response to society's needs and its commitment to humanitarian service.
9. The curriculum includes courses in art, music, literature, and philosophy. Additionally, nursing content is approached using a humanities perspective.
10. Policies, guidelines, and programs of study are formulated in ways that provide for flexibility and accessibility in order to respond to the needs of the nontraditional student.
11. Course construction and teacher–student interactions are forged in ways that acknowledge the adult nature of the learner.
12. Graduate schools on the master's and/or doctoral level offer courses in nursing education with an emphasis on both clinical expertise and educative teaching skills.
13. Faculties' development needs are met by employing full-time faculty/staff development personnel to enable faculty to maintain their clinical and teaching expertise.
14. National accreditation and state-approval mechanisms rest on research-based indicators of excellence that are not related to a curriculum paradigm.
15. Practice settings must change so that they are hospitable places for nurses to exercise the new ways of being that are characteristic of the substantively different professional graduates of the new curricula.

editions, eased up somewhat from the rigidity of the behaviorist paradigm, they have not altered in the de facto criteria. The de facto criteria are those that, in fact, are used by the site visitors in their efforts to verify, clarify, and amplify. The de facto criteria are also used by boards of review in determining the merit of programs. These criteria still tend to be strongly behaviorist-paradigm related. This may be due to such factors as:

1. The orientation of visitors and new board members
2. The pairing of experienced visitors with new ones so that socialization into the process overrides orientation and real criteria
3. The staggering of board membership so that an entirely new board is not possible, therefore old traditions die hard
4. The explanatory materials for accreditation criteria that may enhance the idea that paradigm-related criteria are still very much in force.

These paradigm-required products of curriculum development that are so revered by state approval and accreditation requirements are: a philosophy, conceptual framework, or at least concepts and threads; measurable/behavioral objectives for program, level, course, and units; a required program of study; clearly outlined content that accomplishes the objectives; and evaluation strategies that measure students' ability to meet the required behaviors specified in the objectives. It is clear that there are inherent obstacles in nursing which prevent any changes in paradigm. Until this is altered, all of our revolution is rhetoric, for no one will jeopardize state approval even if he or she is willing to forego national accreditation.

Therefore, the fourteenth indicator of success is the establishment of criteria for state approval and national accreditation of schools of nursing that stress research-based indicators of good schools of nursing and are paradigm-free.

Faculty Preparation and Development

There is a popular belief that graduate level nursing programs should no longer offer functional specialization on either the master's or the doctoral level. The belief is based upon the assumption that teaching nursing is not unique, and therefore if nursing teachers are interested in education courses, they should take them in schools of education. These same people believe that only clinical specialization is appropriate at the master's level. They also believe that if teachers are clinical specialists, productive researchers, and published, they are ipso facto good teachers.

One of the earmarks of a profession is that is has sanctioned ways to educate for the profession. Nursing has certainly illustrated that, with its institutionalization of the Tyler/behaviorist pradigm. However, anyone who has taken courses in schools of education knows that these courses are primarily geared to elementary and secondary school levels, are based upon nonpractice field norms, and have little relevance for classroom and clinical teaching for nursing. Just having intelligence enough to make some transfer from those levels is not enough. So much of what is said is inappropriate to the practice field of nursing and so much of what is appropriate and needed is not said or known. In fact, so much of what we now teach in nursing education courses does not help teachers struggle with helping students learn things that nurses must learn in order to serve society. These nontangible necessities include finding meanings, using intuition safely, examining assumptions, gaining insights, seeing patterns, recognizing significance and implications, being caring and concerned, being idealistic, making moral and ethical commitments, building a background of paradigm experiences, identifying as a professional nurse, inquiring into the nature of things, being creative, strategizing, thinking critically, and knowing about power, its use, control and limits. Whatever teacher education we have must help teachers learn to teach these things. My concept of the new age curriculum development paradigms rests upon an altered role of the teacher—one in which the teacher is an expert nurse and an expert learner who knows how to help others become expert nurses and learners.

Further, we have long accepted the fact that health care agencies must have staff development departments with full-time persons employed as teachers of the staff. As educators, we have assumed that we do not need this and that the occasional workshop or meeting suffices to keep us up to date. That time must pass. Faculty must consistently have access to a colleague-teacher who helps plan and furnish an organized and orderly curriculum in both nursing and educational content so that faculty stay on the cutting edge of expertise and knowledge. In turn, faculty need to have a trusted colleague who helps them change or maintain the roles of teaching through simulation, inquiry, and dialogue.

These ideas lead us to two criteria for success of the revolution: graduate schools on the master's and/or doctoral level offer courses in nursing education with an emphasis on both clinical expertise and educative teaching skills; and faculties employ full time faculty/staff development personnel to enable educators to maintain their clinical and teaching expertise.

Alienation in the Health Care System

If the revolution is a success, and I believe it will be, the graduates of professional programs will have characteristics of professionals, meaning that they will be creative, critical thinkers, ethically astute, professionally autonomous, independent, and collegial in their relationships. These characteristics do not make for good institutional employees. Hospitals are showing the strain of too few nurses and too many slots to fill. Nursing seems to be taking the brunt of the criticism for not graduating enough students. This is not a nursing problem, it is an industry problem.

One of the most severe problems of the industry is that it has become mega-bureaucracy with more of an eye for profits than for people. Nurses traditionally are of the proletariat and identify with the people. They see large numbers of the population without health care coverage, they see creaking and straining in the system from cost to insurers and government, and they see themselves treated as employees without privileges instead of knowledgeable professionals.

Due to the shifts in the health care scene which I mentioned at the beginning of the chapter, there are increasingly more people being cared for in the home. Somewhere I have heard that home health care is the largest growing industry in the United States and I have no reason to doubt it, though I cannot document it. One solution is that professional nurses move out of hospitals into home health where they traditionally have more room for creativity and autonomy. Yet, we cannot abandon those who are the most ill, the most vulnerable, the least able to care for themselves, and the most needy. Professional nurses must remain in hospitals as well as move to home health agencies and nursing homes. To do that we must make health care agencies more hospitable to professional nurses. Now is the time; times of acute shortages are times of change. Now is the time to commence massive negotiations with hospitals, nursing homes, and home health agencies for basic shifts in their attitudes and policies about nurses and to enlist their aid in altering educational practices and state nursing acts regarding the constraints on both education and practice.

My fifteenth and last criterion for success of the paradigm shift in nursing education is that practice settings must change so that they are hospitable places for nurses to exercise the new ways of being that are characteristic of the substantively different professional graduates of the new curricula.

CONCLUSION

These criteria are rough, but for the most part they hit at the heart of the revolution. They point toward the significant and substantive changes that must occur if this revolution is to succeed. I would like them used as a working paper, to be altered and refined and ultimately used to help map the revolution.

We cannot only meet, talk, and write papers; we must organize for change. The National League for Nursing has already formed an informal central planning group whose mission is to establish goals for the revolution. This group, or another similar group, needs to form task forces, each assigned to a separate criterion. These task forces must then plan and execute a national effort to attack the problems and issues relevant to meeting the criteria. Without such an effort our revolution will be slipshod, bloody, self-destructive to nursing, without rigor, and unresponsive to society's needs. We must form a coalition in common cause to improve nursing on behalf of the people we serve.

I end with this thought: (Bevis, 1988)

> There is a compelling splendor about both teaching and nursing that demand the highest forms of endeavor, for their ends are linked to the magnificent miracle of human thought and the quality of human life. They have a common core of caring about the human condition and an obligation to its improvement that confers a radiant beauty on the meanest of tasks in their service. They are a societal trust. And, for those who combine these two tasks into the teaching of nursing, there is a moral commitment to society's needs that requires industrious constancy in improving care so that this trust will be steadfastly and excellently honored. It is to this trust that our revolution is dedicated. (p. 1)

REFERENCES

Benner, P. (1984). *From novice to expert: Excellence and power in clinical nursing practice.* Menlo Park, CA: Addison-Wesley.

Bevis, E. (1982). *Curriculum building in nursing: A process.* St. Louis: Mosby.

Bevis, E. (1988). Teacher as educator: Some directions for faculty development. In E. Bevis & J. Watson (Eds.), *A new direction for curriculum development for professional nursing: A paradigm shift from training to education.* Unpublished manuscript.

Boyd, C. O. (1988). Phenomenology: A foundation for nursing curriculum. In *Curriculum revolution: Mandate for change* (pp. 65–87). New York: National League for Nursing.

Diekelmann, N. (1987). *Alternate models for professional nursing education: new approaches for nursing curriculum development.* Unpublished manuscript.

Diekelmann, N. (1988). Curriculum revolution: A theoretical and philosophical mandate for change. In *Curriculum revolution: Mandate for change* (pp. 137–157). New York: National League for Nursing.

Felton, G. M., & Parsons, M. A. (1984). *The effect of education on the ability to resolve ethical/moral dilemmas.* Columbia, SC: Unpublished paper.

Huebner, D. (1966). Curriculum language and classroom meanings. In *Language and meaning.* Washington, DC: The Association for Supervision and Curriculum Development.

Levin, D. (1983). The poetic function in phenomenological discourse. In W. McBride & C. Schrag (Eds.), *Phenomenology in a pluralistic context.* Albany, NY: State University of New York Press.

Moccia, P. (1988). Curriculum revolution: An agenda for change. In *Curriculum revolution: Mandate for change* (pp. 53–64). New York: National League for Nursing.

Munhall, P. (1988). Curriculum revolution: A social mandate for change. In *Curriculum revolution: Mandate for change* (pp. 217–230). New York: National League for Nursing.

Rest, J. (1979). Manual for the defining issues test: An objective test of moral judgment (rev. ed.). Minneapolis: University of Minnesota.

Sakalys, J., & Watson, J. (1985). New directions in higher education: A review of trends. *Journal of Professional Nursing* (September-October), 293–294.

Tanner, C. (1988). Curriculum revolution: The practice mandate. In *Curriculum revolution: Mandate for change* (pp. 201–216). New York: National League for Nursing.

Watson, J. (1985). *Nursing: Human science and human care: A theory of nursing.* Norwalk, CT: Appleton-Century-Crofts.

Watson, J. (1988). Curriculum in transition. In *Curriculum revolution: Mandate for change* (pp. 1–8). New York: National League for Nursing.

10

Curriculum Reconceptualization: Integrating the Voices of Revolution

Patricia Moccia, PhD, RN

I'd like to begin by suggesting specific concrete steps we must take for this revolution to move forward.

- First, change the power relationships in nursing education, the nursing profession, systems of health care delivery, and higher education. (Indeed change the power relationships in society and in our communities.)
- Begin to change the power relationships by changing our relationship to students and to faculty colleagues, changing our approach to the teaching–learning exchanges that are "the stuffing" of nursing education, changing our attitudes toward it all.
- Change our minds about power, students, control and domination, and nursing and health care.
- Finally, I would like to ask that you consider that "we are them." I will ask you to claim your own voices, your own projects, your own power relationships. Reclaim what has been taken from you, reclaim the teaching–learning interactions and change them toward autonomy and responsibility for both student and teacher, toward a sharing and empathetic relationship, toward health and wholeness and healing.

This chapter will address the theme: "The Curriculum Reconceptualized" and attempt to call our attention to the task of "Integrating the Voices of Revolution." I am hoping that after reviewing the presentations in this book and listening to the discussions, questions, and comments, we will somehow be able to hear what has been said, find the patterns of our voices, hear the themes of our concerns. If all of this is accomplished we can explore them together again, and in the process push our discussions to the next phase, expand the limits of our discourse in our ongoing search for the meaning and understanding of our work, the meaning and understanding of these life projects we've chosen in nursing education.

Capsulizing all of this has not been an easy assignment, not one of my snap projects. Some of the difficulty is that I am not, and hope never to be, comfortable with the presumptive arrogance of knowing what the collective "we" means to be saying. More than my personal discomfort though, the task has been made difficult by what I think I've been hearing—our voices make me uncomfortable. The possibilities of revolution, with all of its blood and turmoil; renaissance, with its historical oppression of women and exalted class discrimination; or maintenance of the status quo and accepting it complacently are all quite disturbing.

I ask you to consider seriously that it is this discomfort that we must address if what I thought to be the aims of this revolution are to be advanced. If this revolution is to happen, then all of us will have our comfort disturbed in an infinite number of ways, places, and instances.

The word revolution *should* make us uncomfortable. There are legitimate fears and concerns that accompany any discussions of whether or not to join the revolution; whether or not to continue with what we have begun; and if so, then how. I ask you to consider these points: (a) the tendency to prefer comforting voices over those that disturb, (b) the conservative rather than revolutionary effect of such a tendency, and (c) whether or not the voices we are hearing reflect the comfort over discomfort choice and so echo a conservative rather than revolutionary force. In other words, the questions I ask you to consider are:

- Do the voices we hear comfort us or make us uneasy?
- What do the voices of our revolution sound like?
- Are the voices we hear the voices we hope to be sounding?

WHAT ARE THE VOICES WE HEAR? AND DO THEY COMFORT OR DISTURB US?

Many of our colleagues hear our voices calling for revolution; hear of these conferences and are excited by the possibilities. "Are there really others talking about change? Are there really nurse colleagues calling for a revolution?" Other colleagues fearful of change, fearful of the unknown, or fearful of both, disclaim us without even hearing what we are saying. Still others are interested, but cynical, and perhaps a bit world weary having lived through promises of change before. They believe that we're saying nothing new, or that the changes we are asking for are not really as revolutionary as we proclaim. Still others listen out of a suspicious concern that there might be some information about accreditation criteria or trends in interpretation which could be useful in helping them tinker with the curriculum here and there, and learn a few new buzzwords to sprinkle in their philosophies and course outlines—letting the site visitors know that their programs are relevant and responsive.

Our voices have been bold and loud and in some ways quite audacious. We have simply pronounced there to be a curriculum revolution. We have gathered the papers of last year's meeting and produced them in a book for mass distribution. We have conducted a national invitational campaign to bring us together to talk of revolution. And we have come together in open forums to make a revolution happen and to plan the stages of a revolutionary campaign.

What kind of revolution can this be, though, that is sponsored by the National League for Nursing? What kind of revolution is conducted under bright lights and in full display? What kind of revolution meets once a year? What kind, when people can foresee relatively unchanged power relationships after the revolution has come and gone?

The contemporary poet Gil Scott-Heron (1970, 1988) tells us in his song that the "revolution will not be televised. . . . that the revolution will be live." Yet we are audiotaping it and selling these tapes for profit. What kind of revolution can this be when the sons and daughters of privilege in this world design the revolution? For that is what we, the educated elite of the nursing profession, have become. We enjoy a position of privilege through the highly produced, determined, and controlled advantage of our education and professional status, and through the equally artificial advantage that accompanies the position that the United States strives so hard to maintain in the world. And now we use that privilege to entertain ourselves with words of revolution.

Can our work as educators who have come together to make a curriculum revolution be compared with the American revolution; or with revolutions in France, Russia, Mexico, China, Cuba, and the Philippines? Are our lives similar to those of Steven Biko who was tortured and killed in South Africa; of political women who have disappeared in the military dictatorships of Chile and Brazil? Can we compare ourselves to the people in Nicaragua, or to Assata Shakur imprisoned in the United States? Does our revolution have anything in common with that of the black and brown "Women of Brewster Place," or the struggles of our own mothers to create love and caring within patriarchal systems, or the battles of our own sisters who seek spaces where it's safe to love first themselves and then one another?

No, this is not the same use of the word revolution. Not if we judge ourselves by the voices we hear—for the voices we hear are dangerously close to speaking of a revolution that has been trivialized, objectified, and commodified like "revolutionary mascara," "revolutionary new cake mix," or "revolutionary new design." This revolution we have marketed, this revolution we have written about, taped, bought, and sold, is not the revolution of revolutionaries. These voices comfort us where the revolutionaries would disturb; these voices will be heard for a short time and dropped into dead space where the revolutionaries will echo; these voices will fade where the revolutionaries will endure.

WHAT DO THE VOICES OF OUR REVOLUTION SOUND LIKE?

Listen closely to the voices that are sounded but yet unheard, to the voices we hope to be speaking. These are the voices connected to the revolution of revolutionaries. Listen, as the feminist poet Adrienne Rich (1979) urges, to the silences for what they tell us, for the voices unheard are the voices of our revolution. The disturbing and unsettling voices within our educator souls that we rush to quiet before they bubble up and explode from our lips are demanding to be heard, as are the voices within our educator spirits that make us so uneasy we only dare to whisper them to our most trusted friends in the privacy of our friendship, swearing them to public secrecy. The voices in our educator passions are debating each other in whispers: Be careful. Go easy. Be brave. Don't be scared. Do it!

Even the surest among us questions what exactly it is we should be doing. The voices you speak over dinner, while shopping; the voices of our passions, our visions, our idealism; the voices that beg themselves for direction are all asking the same question. The passionate and plaintive voices that disturb rather than comfort are our voices, the voices of our revolution.

What is this revolution to which we keep referring? This is another question we have been currently asking and it is the same question asked over 50 years ago by the Russian writer and revolutionary Eugeni Zamyatin. Zamyatin was a key figure in the Russian revolution, but was one of the few Soviet writers who refused to compromise the promise of that revolution to what he took to be Lenin's premature assumption of supreme power. In fact he denounced the Soviet State in 1925 when he stated simply: "Then I was a Bolshevik, now I am not a Bolshevik." In his essay, "On Literature, Revolution and Entropy," Zamyatin (1924) writes:

> Ask the question point blank: What is revolution? You get a variety of replies. . . . Two dead, dark stairs collide with a deafening but unheard

> crash and spark into life a new star—that's revolution. A molecule breaks loose from its orbit, invades a neighboring atomic universe, and gives birth to a new chemical element—that's revolution.

In another context, revolution is the attempt to free people and their institutions through radical political, social, and economic change, so by it's very definition, a revolution disturbs rather than comforts. It overturns relationships of power. It redistributes power. Zamyatin tells us:

> No revolution, no heresy is comfortable and easy. Because it is a leap, it is a rupture of the smooth evolutionary curve, and a rupture is a wound, a pain. But it is a necessary wound. Most people suffer from hereditary sleeping sickness, and those who are sick with this ailment (entopy) must not be allowed to sleep, or they will go to their last sleep, the sleep of death.

If the revolution of which we speak is to create something new, then it must rupture, wound, and inflict pain. The voices of such a revolution are the disquieting ones we've spoken but have yet to hear. They are the voices we mumble to ourselves, which are often painful to speak, but are nonetheless necessary to hear, lest we succumb to the sleep of death.

How many of our curriculum committees can be described the way Zamyatin described his colleagues:

> This same sickness is common to artists and writers. They go contentedly to sleep in their favorite artistic form which they have devised, then twice revised. They do not have the strength to wound themselves, to cease to love what has become dear to them. They do not have the strength to come out from their lived-in, laurel-scented rooms, to come into the open air and start anew.

Do we have the strength to give up the curricula forms we have come to know so well? Can we let go of curricula which have been revised to include every last subject that we can possibly squeeze into our credit loads? After we have figured out how to redesign our curricula to include research; public policy; economics; legal, ethical, and cultural issues; gerontology; critical care; home care; management; leadership; assertiveness; nursing history; feminism; critical theory; nursing theories; and marketing, will we be able to give them up? After we have revised them like Zamyatin's artists and revised our revisions still again, can we let them go? That is one of the questions voiced but yet unheard.

And there is still another question voiced over these last days, one even more fundamental in both its query and implications. What is the true meaning of this word, revolution? In her essay, "Power and Danger:

Works of a Common Woman," Adrienne Rich offers an alternative word and an alternative meaning when she says: "For many of us the word "revolution" itself has become not only a dead relic . . . but a key to the deadendness of male politics. . . . When we (meaning feminists) speak of TRANSFORMATION, we speak more accurately out of a vision of a process which will leave neither surfaces or depths unchanged."

In Sister Rosemary's voice, our revolution is a continuing process in which we ask ourselves essential questions again and again, knowing that no answer can ever be considered final. The voices of our revolution are voices of such continual transformation. Calling for changes in our vision, these are spoken but unheard voices that celebrate process; that would have us look to the form and substance of our relationships; that would have us transform those relationships from being concerned with domination and control to nurturing and nourishing the connections and interdependencies among people and between people and nature; that not only wound as Zamyatin tells us they must, but also heal the wound as Rich tells us. These are voices that transform our lives.

At this point we should ask ourselves to consider seriously whether we are ready to commit ourselves to transformation. Are we able to let go of the power relationship we enjoy with our curricula and with our students—the relationship that legitimates our daring to determine what a student should know and, therefore, what they should not attend to. The position that allows us to proscribe what a curriculum ought look like.

The unspoken voices of our revolution are asking that we consider seriously, as Ellen Fahy asks of us, the ideology of our curricula. What kind of country do we live in, what are the values of a valueless curriculum? Consider whether we are ready to relinquish the illusion we have created, built, and sustained—the illusion that we can dominate and control everything—students, other faculty, the curricula, the curriculum committee, nature.

Consider, as Carol Lindeman has, how nursing practice has changed; how the rationing of health care and nursing education changes the demands on nursing education and the nursing imperative. Consider how different should be our ways to share what we know about people, how different would be our clinical experiences, how different our curricula if we recognize the power we exercise over students. Consider, if our silent voices would be heard, that they would be asking us, urging us, imploring us to turn away from content and predetermined end objectives.

The silent voices of our revolution are asking us to embrace our daily work as educators, as process, as creation of a new order, as reverent moments of transformation of the human spirit.

Can we listen to our voices and reconceptualize the curricula as a life project shared by a community committed to the liberation of the human spirit and the building of a social order that would nourish and nurture such freedom? Will we have the strength to give up our positions of privilege, to wound ourselves, to give up what is most dear, to give up our illusions of power and the false comfort we take from these illusions? Are we willing to come into the open air and start anew? These are the questions in our silences, the disturbing rather than comforting voices that are spoken, but unheard—the voices of our revolution, of our transformation. Zamyatin, again, tells us that "to wound oneself, it is true, is difficult, even dangerous. But to live today as yesterday and yesterday as today is even more difficult for the living."

And, I suggest to you, more dangerous, for if we protect our positions for fear of being wounded (for fear of losing our position of privilege), we will no longer hear even our own voices. They will be stifled, muffled, strangled, and still; and yet another revolution will be betrayed, another transformation cut short.

ARE THE VOICES WE HEAR THE VOICES WE HOPE TO BE SOUNDING?

What would be the experience of curricula so conceptualized? Em Bevis asks us, "How will we know when the revolution is succeeding?" How will we know that it is happening? Who would be our colleagues in *a curricula as life project shared by a community committed to the liberation of the human spirit, committed to building a social order that would nourish and nurture such freedom?*

In his classic essay, "The Moment of Cubism," art critic John Berger (1969) comments and provokes us to look to and listen to each other for the voices of revolution: "If the word revolution is taken seriously, and not merely as an epithet for this season's novelties, it implies a process. No revolution is simply the result of personal originality. The maximum that such originality can achieve is madness; madness is revolutionary freedom confined to the self."

I ask you to look outward from ourselves; look beyond ourselves; somehow break through the perspective we bring as teacher; somehow come to hear the student's voice, as Cynthia Rich asks us to listen to student voices as the voice of colleagues; the voice, as David Allen reminds us, of an autonomous and responsible person. Consider the voices of Nancy Diekelmann, Verle Waters, Gloria Clayton, Clair Martin, Christine Tanner, Lucy Marion, Linda Hardy, and Barbara Hedin as they share with us the lives of students. For it is within the lives of students from which our revolution will come. This will happen not simply from their experiences as students, but from the lives they bring with them to the student–teacher exchange. Listen to the voices of the students, as persons, as agents in their own lives. Remember, as John Brion asks, to listen to students as autonomous and responsible colleagues.

These voices, their unheard voices, express the contradictions of their lives; our unheard voices, the contradictions of our lives. It is these very contradictions from which the power of transformation comes. And so, I suggest to you, that our revolution is advanced and our transformation will happen to the extent that we look to *the shared space between student and teacher as the content of our nursing education.* This shared moment is our reconceptualized curricula; different, admittedly, than what we have known as course work. The content of this revolutionary curricula is our shared lives informed by history and the present; shared lives informed by literature, music, and art; but also affected by the poverty in our streets, varying health conditions, the moral bankruptcy of our leadership, and the threat of nuclear annihilation. Our shared lives reflect the power relationships within society and speak to what reality is, and what the future might be. Curricula, as each of us, comes to exist because and in spite of the realities of separate worlds that speak to each other in the voice of colleagues in the revolution—voices which when joined together are revolutionary voices. Together as colleagues, students and teachers will critically reflect on the power relationships—endemic to all our experiences—that they live through together. Joined together in such a project, in such a curricula, these voices, by the very act of joining, would tell of human interactions and exchanges more caring, more holistic, and simply more healthy than those we've heard of before now.

Such a revolutionary transformation sounds familiar. These could easily be the words of Peggy Chinn. Imagine for a moment that all our teachers had raised their voices calling for love and empowerment, peace and power the way that Peggy does. Imagine that all the voices we heard repeatedly insisted that we attend to the moral context of our work the way that Jean Watson's does. Listen to Peggy's and Jean's voices blend with Adrienne Rich's (1979) who speaks to us of revolution and transformation in her essay, "Writing as Re-Vision."

> . . . there has to be an imaginative transformation of reality, which is in no way passive. And a certain freedom of the mind is needed, freedom to press on, to enter the currents of your thought like a glider pilot, knowing that your motion can be sustained, that the buoyancy of your attention will not suddenly be snatched away. Moreover, if the imagination is to transcend and transform experiences, it has to question, to challenge, to conceive of alternatives, perhaps to the very life you are living at the moment. You have to be free to play around with the notion that day might be night, love might be hate; nothing can be too sacred for the imagination to turn into its opposite or to call experimentally by another name. For writing is re-naming. (p. 43)

The curricula reconceptualized, the voices of revolution and transformation, of wounding and healing, education renamed as a rupture with the past, as the pain we must feel, a revolutionary education that has little if anything to do with content but everything to do with process, an approach to every moment of our lives—all of these are found in the site of our revolution, where our lives will be transformed if at all. Here, within each single moment of a shared experience, is where the revolution will take place.

The transforming voices of our revolution do not speak of either individuals or their worlds, but of the relationship between the two. The transforming voices of our revolution do not speak about what was, or even, solely, about what can be. Rather the transforming voices of revolution shout about the relationships between the two, between what was and what can be. The transforming voices of revolution reveal as many of the real connections between apparently unrelated phenomena as possible; and in the revelation, create new connections, new possibilities.

As we listen beyond the revolutionary voices that are bought and sold, as we listen into the silences, we will hear our revolutionary and transforming voices that disturb us rather than comfort.

— Voices that disturb as they whisper: transform ourselves, explore, know and create anew our relationship to the whole.

— Voices that disturb as they whisper: transform our lives, explore, know and create anew our histories, our present contexts and future possibilities.

— Voices that whisper: transform by refusing to accept as given the separations that divide us from each other, student from teacher, and each from the whole.

— Voices that whisper: transform, connect what has been disconnected.

— Voices that whisper: disrupt relationships of power, domination and submission.

— Voices that whisper: respect and extend the reality of our interdependence.

— Whispering voices that disturb rather than comfort; unheard voices that whispering together transform our lives and heal our pain.

— Voices that speak of paradoxes, of students on strike.

— Voices that speak of pain and call for healing.

— Voices that speak of unspeakable realities and call for revolution.

— Voices that scream for change and call for the transformation of our daily lives and the daily lives of students.

— Voices that tell of the same revolution and the transformation that the contemporary Latin poet Aurora Levin Morales (1981) calls for when she says:

> A revolution capable of healing our wounds.
> If we're the ones who can imagine it
> If we're the ones who dream about it
> If we're the ones who need it most
> Then no one else can do it.
> We're the ones.

Finally, I ask you, urge you, implore you to listen to the unheard voices that whispering together tell of our life projects reconceptualized, of a curriculum reconceptualized. To paraphrase Morales:

> A curriculum capable of healing our wounds.
> If we're the ones who can imagine shared moments of transformation between student and teacher
> If we're the ones who dream about shared moments of transformation between student and teacher
> If we're the ones who need it most
> Then no one else can do it.
> We're the ones.

REFERENCES

Berger, J. (1985). The moment of cubism (1969). In *The sense of sight* (pp. 159–189). New York: Pantheon Books.

Morales, A. L. (1981). . . . And even Fidel can't change that! In C. Moraga & G. Anzaldera (Eds.), *This bridge called my back* (pp. 53–57). New York: Kitchen Table: Women of Color Press.

Rich, A. (1979). *On lies, secrets and silences.* New York: W. W. Norton & Company.

Scott-Heron, G. (1970, 1988). The revolution will not be televised. New York: BMG Music.

Zamyatin, E. (1961). On literature, revolution, and entropy (1924). In P. Blake & M. Hayward (Eds.), *Dissonant voices in Soviet literature.* New York: Harper Colophon Books.